Boundless Bliss

A teacher's guide to

instruction of

restorative yoga

by Chris Loebsack with Tracy Gross &
Jessica Batha

Cover and Content Photos by Brian M. Davis

Cover design by Brian M. Davis

Layout design by Brian M. Davis

Models: Jessica Batha, Tracy Gross, Ernest Batha

ISBN-13: 978-0-9983453-1-4

Dedication &
Acknowledgments

This manual on teaching restorative yoga is offered as an expression of love to all the great teachers, friends and colleagues in my life: past, present and future.

Special thanks to: My parents Chuck and Sue Loebsack, Leigh Ann Stratakos, Jason Nemer, Mary Aranas, Frank Riccobono, Carter Loebsack, Faramarz, Charlotte Kresge, Dr. Richard Pekala, Jason Ray Brown, Carolyn Suddha-Lundeen, Justin Caruso and Corinne Farrell.

This edition would not be possible without the hard work of my colleagues Tracy Gross and Jessica Batha, whose help and additions were invaluable. Along with Bud Batha, they were also the models in the photos throughout the book and on the cover. Thanks to Sara Koresh, Diane Stanton and Katie McHugh-Connelly for policing the grammar and punctuation.

Special thanks to my husband Brian Macrae Davis, Author of The Skye's Eyes, for all of the support in editing, formatting and love that has been poured into this book and into our life together.

With gratitude,

Chris Loebsack

Before engaging in any practice always consult your physician. Yoga practice should complement, but never take the place of medical advice and attention.

Forward

"Damn it!" Red juice ran down my new white blouse. I felt the tears welling up again. It was about the tenth time that week I had lost control of my arm and dribbled something on another clean outfit. I worried that I may end up worse and soon need a child's sippy cup to keep from making a mess of myself. I was sixteen years old when the pain began in my neck, back and arms; I was tired and growing frustrated.

My parents shuttled me from doctor to doctor as I explained that I was having trouble competing that season for my high school swim team. At first, most doctors checked for the usual culprits like a torn rotator cuff or muscle strains, but each visit held less answers than the last. One doctor, acting like my pain was all in my head, decided steroids would be helpful. If 'helpful' means a massive water-weight gain to go along with the pain, then yes he was successful. I was now seventeen, feeling more awkward than ever, and still in constant discomfort. At the end of the list of doctors I landed at a sports medicine clinic where I would hear the word 'fibromyalgia' for the very first time. I was given this medical condition (characterized by widespread pain and joint stiffness) as a diagnosis and told that relief was only possible through the use of pain medications and I should avoid physical activity as it would only aggravate my condition. If I still wanted to swim I would have to learn to live with the pain (doctors still had a lot to learn about fibromyalgia).

I was determined not to let something that seemed so foreign to me to keep me down. I was still in pain. Always. But, I muffled my complaints. I took on every activity I could think of as a distraction. I discovered that the busier I was the less the pain was noticeable, while periods of inactivity were filled with pain. Consequently, in the years between the end of high school and college I averaged about five hours of sleep an evening. I was becoming the model type-A personality. I had grown into a fine young, aggressive, and dependable workaholic.

Things came to a head in 1994 when I began developing a series of bladder infections. The final bladder infection took hold and dove deeper into my kidneys. I was stubborn and didn't want to go to the hospital because I would miss my dance recital that season. A few hours later my mom found me lying on the bathroom floor and with a mother's patience said, "Are you ready to go to the hospital now?"

After the hospital, I was feeling better and ready to get right back to my busy schedule. My doctor gave me a yearlong set of antibiotics and sent me on my way. It boggles my mind now to think that any doctor would put anyone on an antibiotic for a year! I shudder now to think of the effects on my immune system. At the time, however, armed with my bottle of pills I jumped back into work.

Shortly after the resumption of my hectic schedule, deep depression sank in. I assumed it was from a recent emotional break with a boyfriend, but as time passed I couldn't get out of my funk. As it turned out I was suffering from sleep deprivation. I would fall asleep each night and try to get six to seven hours of sleep, but would actually wake up every fifteen to twenty minutes. I was completely devoid of REM sleep which is essential for healing. I was, in essence, torturing myself. A few more bottles of pills (this time anti-depressants) and I was once again off and running, this time feeling devoid of emotional highs and lows. I was numb.

Despite the obstacles I found in my path, my high school and college years were nevertheless fun and rewarding. However I now realize that my coping strategies were often as much of a hindrance as they were a help. I wish I had known how to take better care of myself so I could have participated more fully in my own experiences. I know better now!

During my last years of college, I was introduced to yoga by my mother. She thought it would be nice for us to have some bonding time since I was always so busy. Jiavana Skolnick was the teacher. She was a shorter and stout woman with curly hair and a kind face. I felt relaxed almost immediately by the setting in the room. There were a few simple candles, soft piano music in the background and a faint hint of lavender in the air. Mom and I sat on our mats. After class I wasn't sure where the hour and a half went. I believe I slept through most of it. I felt pretty rested. I felt good.

I hated the way my "medicine" made me feel so I decided to

throw it out. Instead, I tried to get to a yoga class whenever I could. It would be years, though, before I would practice with any consistency. I fell right back into my old patterns. Work more, feel less.

My consistent practice began in 2001 when I met Jennifer Logosso, 500hr ERYT of Sundari Yoga in Stroudsburg, at a partner yoga workshop. I dragged my friend Bob along (who was always a good sport) as we playfully explored some poses. Jenn walked over with a smile and said, "You should come to my studio and see me. I could help you a lot with your practice." I showed up at Sundari Yoga a few months later and began taking classes daily. She was correct.

For the first time in years, any soreness I felt was from using my muscles, not from mystery pain. My joints began to experience freedom and spaciousness. I was getting stronger each day. Seeing my dedication, Jenn encouraged me to train as a teacher. I laughed, thinking, "No way." I was happy on my mat and didn't want to teach. Jenn politely ignored me and stated that she really needed a teacher to take over some classes. She knew I was finding loose change under my car seat to pay for classes and offered to train me in an exchange for teaching at her studio. If I didn't like it after I paid off my training I would be in the clear. It was the offer that changed my life.

I completed the Sundari Yoga 200hr training program and began teaching immediately. The funny thing to me was that I enjoyed teaching as much or more than my personal practice. I was teaching four classes a week in addition to the 50-60hrs a week I was working as a bar and restaurant manager. I remained completely dedicated to my personal practice. This, again, didn't leave time for much else.

I knew I needed a break but wanted to continue my yoga study. I used my vacation days to go to Kripalu and study Restorative Yoga with Carolyn Suddha Lundeen. I fell back into the bliss of cushions, comfort and stillness. This was such a welcome sweetness and diversion from my normal Ashtanga practice. After years of fighting my body, I surrendered. Despite my consistent yoga practice my busy schedule kept me stressed. I knew that if I didn't listen to my body I was going to crash and burn. I steadily worked more gentleness into my routines. I cut back my work schedule. I shifted my attitude toward my pain and I began to feel calmer.

Each year, I would use my vacation to continue my yoga education. In 2006, I expanded my practice with Dharma Yoga 500HR and AcroYoga teacher trainings. AcroYoga lead me to the gift of Thai massage and additional therapeutic practices that continue to be a part of the larger focus of my current work.

I have not had a fibromyalgia flare up in years. Restorative Yoga taught me how to be still and listen to my body. In those moments, I found the courage to let go. There is a deeper awareness of the feeling of each breath and how that breath moves within me. I now sleep soundly a solid seven and a half hours a night. My new motto is 'work less, feel more.'

In 2010, I was invited to spend three weeks with two of my greatest teachers, Jason Nemer and Jenny Sauer-Klien for the Level

2 AcroYoga teacher training. What might really surprise many, since AcroYoga is often known for its more elaborate acrobatic endeavors, is that the mantra of our training became LIFE BALANCE! It was a loving reminder that past habits do not have to set the patterns for our future choices. Instead, we can choose a path that brings us fulfillment, joy and love. I am still sometimes wavering on the line between my workaholic tendencies and the new embodiment of *sukha* (good space). However, I constantly keep in mind that each moment is a chance to experience life fully and live with greater ease.

I began writing this manual in 2007 as an exercise to organize all of the scattered information from various classes and workshops that I had acquired over a decade of study. This text is a collage of numerous inspirations from many talented teachers and students alike. I am sure that over the years it will continue to build and grow. Life and learning are amazing gifts and I can't wait to see what is in store for me next. My wish is that this text will help teachers and students find the stillness and ease they need to let go of anything that no longer serves them.

In 2017, I was excited to open this manual to collaboration with Jessica Batha and Tracy Gross. While there have been other revisions and additions, this edition is extremely special. Jessica and Tracy each bring years of knowledge, a fresh perspective and incredible joy to the work. It is an honor to collaborate with these amazing women and we hope you enjoy our offering.

In service and with gratitude I bow to you. ~ Chris Loebsack

Table of Contents

Section 1:

Foundations of the Practice

"By means of microscopic observation and astronomical projection, the lotus flower can become the foundation for an entire theory of the universe and an agent whereby we may perceive truth." -**Yukio Mishima**

Restorative Yoga and Deep Relaxation

What is restorative yoga?

Restorative yoga is a style of yoga accessible to anyone at any time to create balance, quiet and restore our bodies and minds to a state of homeostasis. The system uses props and supports that allow the practitioner to hold poses for a longer period of time without strain, promoting deeper relaxation and creating a space for healing. Restorative yoga has a great therapeutic impact during times of stress: illness, injury, pain, and over-scheduled lives. Restorative yoga helps to cultivate a healing environment in the body by balancing the nervous system's optimal energy flow, restoring us at a physical, physiological, energetic and emotional level. Props may include, but are certainly not limited to, blankets, bolsters, chairs, blocks, straps and eye pillows.

What are the Benefits of Restorative Yoga?

- Deep relaxation

- Stress reduction

- Restores balance in body and mind

- Promotes a healthy spine

- Calm and quiet mind

- Balances the nervous system

- Develops qualities of understanding and compassion towards ourselves and others

- Improves sleep quality

Restorative yoga gives balance to the fast paced and overstimulated culture of our modern existence. Slowing down with restorative yoga creates the calm internal environment that gives us the capacity to alleviate physical and mental symptoms caused by stress. Stress, including physical, mental, emotional and environmental stress is the root of disease. Restorative yoga aims to clear the way for deep personal healing. Flow aka *vinyasa* or alignment classes aka *hatha* classes are physically challenging and engage the muscles as a form of exercise in the poses or *asanas*, Restorative yoga is quite the opposite and uses no muscular contraction to hold the poses. The tools often referred to as props support the body fully so that we can increase flexibility gradually in a passive stretch without any strain. The body is then allowed to fully relax into the posture and the many layers of tension we may hold can drift away with breath and time.

Restorative and Yin Yoga: Are They The Same?

On the surface restorative yoga and yin yoga may look very similar. The beauty of both approaches to yoga is that they teach the student to feel, developing a powerful inner awareness. Both restorative and yin yoga cultivate stillness, meditation, and deep awareness, but they access these states in different ways. Both approaches will hold poses for a longer duration, yet how these poses are held and the intensity to which they are held will vary significantly.

In yin yoga, poses are held in a challenging, yet comfortable space for a period of several minutes. The aim of yin yoga is to place an additional stress on the tissues using gravity as a tool for allowing the tissues to release with time. Yin uses a moderate amount of physical stress in the form of static/active or static/passive stretch techniques. Rarely are props incorporated into the yin practice. The goal with yin is to work the connective tissue called fascia, thereby opening up the range of motion and working to increase the general level of flexibility. Yin yoga works deep into the connective tissues and myofascial pathways to activate change at the deepest level. The postures also work to open and free up energy flow, or meridian lines, of the body. The pure intention of yin yoga is to to pay close attention to sensations in the body and mind. In yin yoga we may experience mild to moderate discomfort in a range of possibilities not limited to the physical body. Thoughts and emotions may surface and through a yin practice, we will sit and stay with these sensations for a period of time in order to either change how we feel or learn to approach them with clarity.

Restorative yoga is focused on the restoration of the balance in the nervous system through the use of fully supported postures so the muscles can release and the mind can rest. This helps to restore a stressed, unhealthy body or injured body, to rebound and return to a healthy, uninjured and unstressed state. Restorative yoga asks that we release the thoughts, triggers and stresses of the mind and body and deeply relax. This means that there is very little effort of any kind during a practice. Restorative uses only static/passive techniques with support for minimal stretch. It is possible receive some yin style benefit from restorative yoga postures as the poses are also held for a longer period of time. In restorative yoga, however the goal is to access tranquility and peace through healing nurturing postures. While in the postures, the body can activate the parasympathetic side of the nervous system, affectionately known as rest and digest mode. The props help the body avoid the physical stress or tensegrity that would otherwise be present in a yin practice. The pure intention of restorative yoga is to find relaxation and to decrease stress at the physical, emotional, mental and energetic levels.

In a nutshell: Restorative yoga heals a body in need of healing. Yin yoga activates change at a very deep level in an already healthy body to increase performance.

For a more thorough explanation of types of stretch, see the section, Working with Stretch and Properties of Skeletal Tissue

Create a Comfortable Practice Space

Restorative yoga requires props as tools to assist the body into the most supported state. You do not have to have everything to have a successful practice, however the more tools you have, the more creative you can be. Here are the basic and most commonly used tools of the practice:

• Some time, when you are not feeling rushed	• 4 Blankets (Wool or Mexican)
• A clean and open space free from distractions	• Bolster (1-2)
• Soothing background music	• 2-4 Blocks
	• 1-2 Straps
	• Folding chair
	• Eye pillow

| | • Yoga mat |
| | • Sandbags |

Dedicating a space in your home for your practice ensures you are more likely to use it. If you don't have to rearrange furniture, de-clutter, and spend precious time thinking about "thinking about it" you simply go to your mat. A designated space can also help you cultivate awareness. You may begin to notice how the light shifts in different seasons, how the colors change from month to month and how your mind greets the same space with new thoughts.

- Dedicate a space just for your practice. Make sure the space is comfortable, clean and uncluttered.

- Unplug from the world and make this time your own. This is your space and time to recharge and renew, so keep it free of distractions. Turn off the TV, computer and phones.

- Set the room temperature. (When you hold poses longer without a good deal of movement you may become chilled.)

- Place a few objects of inspiration in your area.

- Keep your props close at hand so you do not have to break your flow when you need them.

- Ambiance can set the mood of your practice. You may use lights to brighten or dim to set the tone. Use essential oils or soft music. Candles may be soothing, but use them with caution. It is not relaxing or safe to fall asleep during a restorative pose only to wake up to a fire. Creating this sense of ritual can help the body "drop in" to a state of relaxation.

While these points are being applied to a home practice, the should also be considered when teaching restorative yoga in a studio. Most studios have already addressed the first column. If you are going to be teaching restorative yoga, be sure that you have enough props for each of the students attending your class. For this reason, restorative yoga classes often will have a cap on the number of students who are allowed to attend because they can be prop-heavy. In order to ensure that you have enough props for your class, it can be helpful to layout out all of the props you will be using at each of the student's practice spots, that way you are not scrambling mid-class for extra props.

Keys to a Successful Practice

Whether you are preparing for your personal practice or leading a class full of students, these may help you have a successful experience. Once the space is ready for you and you have all props and tools that you desire for your practice, it is time to begin. The restorative practice, or any yoga practice, will be most beneficial if we can approach it with a positive attitude and a sense of benevolent curiosity. The practice can cultivate self-love and patience which is more important than the actual shapes we make with our bodies.

- Approach your practice with "metta"; loving-kindness.

- Make sure everything feels GOOD.

- Look for supportive alignment and comfort.

- Do not beat yourself up if things do not go as planned.

- Be willing to change your plan if something else feels better for you.

- For some students it is helpful to keep a practice log.

- A good way to stay on track is to make your practice the first part of your day or at the same time each day.

- Take your time. Do not rush the transition between poses. Move mindfully and take time to reflect.

- Whenever possible take your time before entering the regular activities of the day so you can ease back into the normal energy of life.

Guiding Students into Poses

In music, the scales are the thread of all creative expression. The taste and style of sound may be widely varied, but the skilled musicians are all playing the same notes. From the strong foundation and practice of the scales, the musician can then find the freedom to explore rhythm, tempo and musical texture. The most profound musical scores and creativity have emerged from the solidity of structure. Similarly, the most advanced educators teach the basic material with impeccable form and precision. When a teacher fully embodies the foundations of form, (s)he has the freedom to create.

Look at the classroom in front of you. Really look and see and feel the individuals in front of you. You are accepting the honorable role of service. Your position is to create a container where students may explore their own experience with safety, support and guidance. This is a student-centered classroom and as such should be free of your personal expectations and ego. It is not important that the student form a specific shape of a particular posture with his/her body. Rather as a teacher, can you guide him/her into the expression of the posture that supports his/her body and mind safely while exploring the curious edges of his/her practice? In this way you can begin to look beyond the mass of the class toward each individual.

Teacher is just one of the roles that you will express as a yoga educator. Some characterizations you will choose to take on and others will be appointed to you even when you don't realize it. You may find yourself viewed as a parent, friend, spiritual adviser, doctor, lover, business person and more. When you step into the role of the teacher you carry a great responsibility. You may be surprised by some of the titles listed above. Remember we are discussing how students may perceive you and the information you present, not implying that you are actually taking these roles. Simply knowing how your words and actions as a teacher may influence others will hopefully bring you to a place of consistent mindfulness and skillful action. We would highly recommend continuing study in ethics to support your continuing education as a human and as a teacher.

Important Points About Teaching Your Restorative Class

- **Demonstrate:** Working with props can be confusing to students. Many students rely heavily on the visual cues to guide them into supported postures.

  - Make sure you are in a location where the students can see you.

  - Make eye contact

  - Make sure the action points are visible

- Vary the side of the body you demo on to keep your own body open and safe

- **Explain how the posture works:**
  - Name the posture
  - Carefully present the foundations
  - Break down the pose, step by step
  - Don't be afraid to repeat yourself (students learn by repetition)
  - Use an authentic voice
  - Use an appropriate volume
  - Cue specific points
  - Cue the inhale/exhale

- **Offer verbal guidance:** *Tune in to the art of imparting knowledge, in this case verbal cueing.* After you have shown them, students will still need verbal cues to help them place the props.
  - Use simple and concise language, not too much information and nothing extra.
  - If you are using a theme in class this is a nice space to drop in a few gems.
  - Know the difference between cues that will re-instruct, correct, and refine and when to use each wisely.
  - Give verbal cues to get into the posture, when students have settled give them a breath cue, let them know how

long they will be in the posture, guide a deep breath before cueing the release out of the posture.

- **Observe:** Allow time for students to adjust their props for maximum comfort and release.

  - Develop the habit of keen awareness and noticing and attentively watching.

  - Find a clear space in the classroom where you can see all, or most of the students.

  - Reposition and move around the room to see it from all angles.

  - Observe from the ground up and look for balanced actions.

  - Read students' facial expressions and body cues.

  - Watch for clothing bunching, skin pinching and postural collapses. These might indicate discomfort.

  - Correct or cue based on observation, avoid instruction-by-rote or random cues. Keep it fresh and relevant to the individual or group.

  - Stay connected and be creative: The needs will vary from student to student. Encourage patience and release with both verbal and tactile cues.

- **See the unseen:** Restorative yoga can be challenging. The body may look "quiet," but the mind may still be restless.

- **Silence:** The space created by silence offers the opportunity for students to feel observe and fully experience their

14

journey.

Qualities of a Restorative Yoga Teacher

The most well-received classes are the ones where students feel amazing. The connection students make to their teacher will largely determine how students perceive the class. Feeling safe and welcomed goes a long way in any set of material.

- **Positivity:** Take the optimistic approach. Always look for the best in yourself and others.

- **Compassionate/non-judgment:** Every class provides only a small window into the world of each student. Each individual has an intricate life history with his/ her own journey of sorrows and joys that are not ours to judge. Invite connection and trust by creating an atmosphere of compassion. You can be a witness to another's journey, but as restorative teachers we are positive facilitators of that journey, not doctors or counselors. Always approach a student from a place of support and guidance. We do not "fix" students. If a student approaches you with a concern beyond the scope of your training or an issue that falls into the category of another licensed field, give them a referral to an appropriate source for additional help.

- **Full presence:** Teachers should be aware of what is going on with an ever-present eye on the class.

- **Firm but gentle:** Be confident in your adjustments, but without force.

- **Patience (never rush):** Keep a steady flow to the class without hurry or pause. Keep in mind the flow of a class can change. Keep a timepiece near and be prepared to omit or add a pose as necessary so you may leave time for a complete savasana.

- **Support:** If a posture is not working for a student they may get frustrated. Find a way to re-support. If needed, change to a different posture to suit the student. This practice is about comfort and healing not keeping up with what other students are doing. Passive postures can evoke uncomfortable emotions for a myriad of reasons. Any emotions a student may have been suppressing throughout the day—fear, frustration, sadness, anxiety—are likely to come to the forefront of the mind once the body begins to relax. It is worth noting that whatever comes up for students is what comes up. We as teachers do not have to project an emotion; i.e. "you may feel sadness in this hip-opener".

- **Receptivity:** Be available and approachable to your students. Students should always feel welcome and safe in your presence.

Set Up, Warm Up, Conclusion

Create the perfect container so that the participants have a complete experience from beginning to end.

Set Up

- Make sure all props and necessary items are available for your students ahead of time. It will be distracting to the students' relaxation process to have to get up and retrieve an extra prop. Create a prop list for students to begin with.

- Check the room's temperature.

- Set ambiance: remove clutter, address lighting, music or silence.

- Prepare your personal space. Take time to ground yourself before students enter to ensure you are able to remain present with them at all times. Wash your hands, meditate for a few minutes, you set the tone and the experience for your students.

- Set a tone or theme to guide the students' experiences.

- Have your syllabus of desired poses and inspirational directions at hand.

- Let students know that they should use the restroom prior to entering their mat space.

- Offer anyone water that did not come with their own.

- Breathe. Maintaining steady, unlabored breath while assisting and adjusting students as this can sometimes be challenging, especially in a large class.

Warm up

- A brief tutorial at the top of class is helpful to those new to restorative yoga.

- Vocal cues begin the moment you are in front of the class.

- Decide how you want to handle hands-on adjustments. Give them permission to opt-out if they wish.

- Let the class know what to expect and that you are there to make their restorative practice successful.

- Take some time at the beginning for some gentle asana or joint mobilizations to prepare the body for long periods of stillness. For instance, if you are working a sequence of seated postures you may want to warm up the hips and hamstrings.

Conclusion

- Invite students to take their time and move mindfully after class. Remind students to drink some water.

- You have just created a moment for students to be nurtured. Tune into *seva* (selfless service) and clean the room. The group cleanup process can turn chaotic, undermining the relaxing work they have just done. Cleaning up after the class can become part of a teacher's meditation.

Getting Comfortable:

"Good enough" or "alright" is not OK. Strive for total comfort.

Students (or yourself in your home practice) will be surrendering to these postures often for 5, 10 or 15 minutes, so the slightest discomfort upon setup will quickly magnify itself. It is impossible to relax if you are not entirely comfortable. As teachers we need to be aware not only of the verbal cues that let us know to readjust a student.   We must also be vigilant and watchful for body movements such as fidgeting or constant shifting. Some students may not tell you when they are feeling uncomfortable. Notice all the details. If we remain present we can help guide them back into a safe and happy comfort zone. Support all the spaces so students can truly sink into the props and avoid a, "Princess and the Pea" dilemma. When you teach a class you will often ask a student, "How does that feel?" Often you will receive answers such as, "Alright", "Good enough" or "OK." All of these are unacceptable. We are looking for answers like "Good", "Great" and "Mmm...". Don't settle for anything less than absolute comfort. Be observant. Are their feet restless? Are they tapping a finger? Are all parts of the body supported? (i.e.: a dangling arm, a suspended foot) Subtle signs can tell us when full release has not been achieved. A student may say they are "OK" and at the same time make a subtle gesture to a particular part of the body. This is a clue to tune into possible discomfort and an opportunity for you to assist.

Be aware that while you may begin to heat up as you move around the room making adjustments and shifting props, your students are either not moving at all or using minimal movement from pose to pose. This means that they will begin to lower their body temperature. Be sure to keep extra blankets on hand to cover students. It is also hard to relax if your toes are cold. Socks may be left on for comfort.

When releasing from one posture and preparing for the next, do NOT rush. Take your time between postures and allow for some soft breathing and personal observation. You can offer cat/cow, extended leg stretches, and moderate movement when moving from one restorative yoga pose to another. Be open to the possibilities, needs, energy, and flow of the class. Some students may fall asleep in some relaxation postures. Keep your voice soft or use a gentle arm stroke to wake them. Never startle a student who has drifted off. They may have really needed that deep rest so do not ruin the moment with jarring motions or loud noise.

Bring your own creativity and personal touch to your students. What are your gifts and talents that make you truly unique?

Meditate on your own unique gifts and implement them into your teaching. Do you play an instrument, sing, aromatherapy, write poetry or are you a certified Reiki practitioner or licensed massage therapist? These are just a few examples of personalizing your classes and bringing your unique gifts to your students. Offering our authentic self is the greatest gift we can give. Offering your authentic self makes you approachable and interesting. It can feel quite vulnerable when you begin to share your gifts, but you will find the rewards to be priceless.

Section 2

The Brain and the Body

"What good is speed if the brain has oozed out along the way?"

- St. Jerome

Stress

Stress finds us on varying levels. We don't have to look for it- it finds us. Whereas "rest" is something we must invite to our lives. We, as a society must initiate rest. We hear the term "stress," often in phrases like, "I'm so stressed out," "I can't take the stress" or "the stress you dish out is giving me gray hair." By definition, stress is a term for the biological response to physical or emotional threats, real or imagined, that bring about mental, physical or emotional strain.[1] These mental, physical and emotional strains can lead to significant health consequences in both the brain and the body. Restorative yoga is a tool for stress management; and it is helpful to be upfront about how challenging restorative yoga actually can be.

Remember that not all stress is negative. We can use appropriate levels of stress to grow in our bodies, hearts and minds. For our purposes in restorative yoga training, we will focus on overcoming negative stressors.

---

1 *The Stress of Life*, Hans Selye, New York, McGraw Hill, 1978

Types of Stress

Environmental/Chemical: Environmental stress is the response of the body and mind to external stimuli. This could be the noise around you, pollution in the air to the medications you take and the foods you eat.

A yogic example is the idea of *saucha* or cleanliness, also described as purity is a personal observance or *niyamas*. This tool of keeping a clean space, clean food and pure environment, helps to reduce environmental/chemical stress.

Physical: Physical stress involves rigorous or strenuous activity. Not all physical stress in negative. Physical exercise will put various stressors on the muscles that can be healthy or unhealthy depending upon the amount time and degree of intensity.

A yogic example is *asana* or the postures which are a part of the 8-limbed practice. In restorative yoga, we are aiming for minimal physical stress.

Mental and Emotional: This type of stress is more internal. Mental/emotional stress is often caused by worrying about situations we cannot control. Typically this stress plays out like a broken record in the mind.

These types of stressors are the very reason that a yoga practice was born. In the Yoga Sutras of Patanjali, a common text on yoga philosophy, Patanjali states in the second line that yoga is to still the patterns of the mind. The space created by the stillness of the restorative practice is a powerful tool to help us overcome a busy mind. Mental chatter is a part of our human condition and the practice of breathing along with the postures will help to calm the nervous system and reduce mental and emotional distress.

Fight or Flight Response

Fight or flight response, also called acute stress response, was first described by Walter Cannon in 1915. His theory states that animals will respond to emotional or physical threats by preparing the body to either stand to fight or move in flight. These two reactions are prompted by the action and release of chemicals in the sympathetic nervous system. When we are in a non-stress or non-emergency state the body can use energy for other biological processes such as healing through rest and digestion.

Restorative poses help balance the sympathetic and parasympathetic nervous system by initiating a relaxation response as we tap into the parasympathetic side of the nervous system or the rest and digest side. The relaxation response is a term used to describe the measurable effects of tapping into the 'rest and digest mode,' or parasympathetic side of the nervous system.

How do we initiate the parasympathetic side of the nervous system and tap into the relaxation response?

- Clear distractions

- Take time to get quiet. We need space for the mind to relax.

- Soften and elongate breathing patterns. You can choose to simply focus on the breath becoming more spacious or use one of a variety of pranayama (directed breathing patterns) to shift the breath rate and depth.

The Nervous System

The nervous system regulates the body's response to internal and external stimulation through a complex system of cells, tissues and organs. In humans the nervous system is composed of brain, spinal cord, nerves, and ganglia. The nervous system is divided into three parts, the Central Nervous System (CNS), the Peripheral Nervous System (PNS), and the Enteric Nervous System (the latter is rarely discussed outside of the medical community and is related to the gastrointestinal tract, the pancreas and gall bladder).[2] We will not be concerned with the Enteric Nervous System for this course.

The Central Nervous System (CNS)

The Central Nervous System (CNS) includes all the nervous system

---

2 HTTP://faculty.washington.edu/chudler/auto.html

elements that are protected by bone. The CNS begins with the brain which is protected by the skull. The skull has tiny spaces between the bones (about the width of a sheet of paper), these are "immovable joints" called sutures. These sutures, in fact, do have micro movement of about 40 microns which is similar to the motion of breathing. This allows for the motion of synovial fluid. The brain pulses about 12 times a minute moving synovial fluid with electrical impulses. The brain, protected by the bones of the skull has an opening at the base for the brain stem and spinal cord which continues on and is then protected by the vertebral bodies.

The Brain

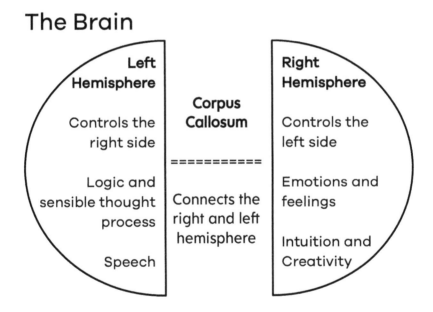

The brain cannot generate new nerves, but the brain can strengthen the connections between nerves. When we use repetition we actually hardwire our receptors. The adage, "old habits die hard," will hold true until you rewire the nervous system response. This is how we develop neuro-muscular memory.

Some of us develop one side more than the other; some of us apply both sides equally. There is no right and wrong, however linking to one side more predominantly than another will influence how we learn, process and retain information. When the right hemisphere and left hemisphere work together there is reason, motivation, compassion and a balance of emotions. The tools of a yoga practice: meditation, pranayama, and asana work at the level of the brain to yoke the benefits of both hemispheres and bring about union and harmony. This unity in thought begins to spill into our daily lives decreasing stress and bringing about contentment.

Peripheral Nervous System (PNS)

The Peripheral Nervous System (PNS) includes all of the nerves radiating from the spine which stem out and are directed into the limbs. The PNS is not under the direct protection of bone cover.

The Autonomic Nervous System

The Autonomic Nervous System is the division of the Peripheral Nervous System (PNS) that controls the involuntary actions of smooth muscle, skin, heart, organs and glands. In this system there are two types of nerves with opposite reactions. One type increases blood pressure and body responses (Sympathetic Nervous System), and the other that decreases blood pressure and slows down the body (Parasympathetic Nervous System).

Sympathetic	Parasympathetic
Fight or flight response aka instinctual responses	Freeze or recover response aka rest and digest mode
Increase heart rate	Decrease heart rate
Decrease digestion	Increase digestion
Pupils dilate	Pupils constrict
Increase in respiration (O2)	Decrease in respiration (O2)
Increase in "smelly" sweat in arms and legs (where they attach to the torso)	Diffuse sweat; full body

This sympathetic state is important as it allows our bodies to react with quick response to danger. However, it can cause stress-related illness if left spinning in high gear for prolonged periods of time. Conversely, trauma can drop an individual into the deepest levels of the parasympathetic side that can leave them feeling numb and unresponsive.

In our culture many individuals are stuck in the sympathetic state due to higher levels of stress and anxiety. During a yoga class, restorative postures and certain pranayama (breathing techniques) allow the body to drop into the parasympathetic state where healing and recovery happen, which can lead to the purging of emotional response. Yoga nidra (yogic sleep) and trance states also dip into the parasympathetic state. We are striving for a condition of homeostasis where there is a balance between the sympathetic and the parasympathetic states. As individuals we try to maintain this mid-range where we do not have extremes on one side or the other.

Restorative yoga brings us the space and time necessary to tap into the parasympathetic side of the nervous system allowing us the time to rest and digest. Supported by the props, the body can release which allows the breath to slow down and the heart rate to calm. In addition to the physical benefits from the relaxation response, we can find tremendous solace in the mind. Restorative yoga becomes an oasis for the body mind and spirit to retreat from our daily stressors.

The Endocrine System

The nervous system carries signals stimulating hormonal information around the body quickly. The effects are immediate and short lived. The endocrine system takes a little longer to get going but the effects will last for hours and even weeks.

Hormones control and regulate:

- Reproduction

- Metabolism and energy balance

- Growth and development

- Body defenses

- General homeostasis and water, nutrient, and electrolyte balance of the blood

Endocrine glands include; pituitary gland in your brain, thyroid gland in your throat, adrenals, pancreas, and gonads. Hormones are produced and released here, but they circulate through your whole body, binding with cells that have the receptors to accept them. Some are more localized and sent to one particular area of the body.

The pituitary makes hormones that signal other hormones to be produced elsewhere (referred to as cascades). It is the mastermind of the endocrine system. The pituitary is connected to the hypothalamus which is the connector of the nervous and the endocrine system. The endocrine system depends on the sensory information taken in from the nervous system to decide which hormones to produce (i.e. baby crying, mammary glands start milk production and secretion). The pituitary is two different glands fused together. The posterior pituitary secretes two hormones made by the hypothalamus; oxytocin (used in contractions in the uterus during pregnancy, milk production, social recognition, pair bonding, orgasms and anxiety), and anti-diuretic hormone (tells the kidneys to retain water). The anterior pituitary produces and secretes many hormones, some of which end up in the thyroid. The thyroid regulates your metabolism, appetite, muscle function, blood pressure, and heart function.

The adrenals are controlled by the pituitary and sit on top of the kidneys. They help control how much salt and water are in your body. They also respond to stress. As soon as the body senses that something dangerous is happening, the nervous system tells the pituitary to secrete adrenocorticotropic hormone (ACTH) which signals the adrenals to make epinephrine (or adrenaline). This tells the organs of the body to do a bunch of different things at once: cut off the blood supply to your digestive system, send blood to your muscles, speed up your heart. Unlike all the other muscles in your body, your heart is controlled by both the nervous and endocrine system. You may notice after a scare that you heart races for a couple of minutes afterward, that is due to the epinephrine from the endocrine system.

The pancreas is the biggest gland in the body. It regulates glucose in the blood which makes cellular respiration. When you eat a cupcake, your pancreas releases insulin (beta cells) to the body to help absorb glucose into the cells. Liver and muscle cells help convert glucose into glycogen for storage and other tissues in the muscle cells called adipose convert glucose into fat. The pancreas also helps out if your blood sugar level is too low. It releases glucagon (through alpha cells) which tells the liver and muscles to start breaking up the glycogen and fat to release the glucose to use as energy.

There are a few endocrine-related imbalances like diabetes and hypothyroidism that occur when there is too little or too much hormone being produced. Hyper is too much and hypo is too little. One of the larger cascades that occurs is in the hypothalamic-pituitary-adrenal-axis or HPA Axis. This interaction controls a lot of your daily processes like digestion, sexuality, immune response and how you handle stress. This is the endocrine system's companion to the sympathetic nervous system, or fight/flight engagement.

Keeping the endocrine system healthy by allowing the body to come down and initiate the relaxation response during restorative yoga creates balance in the body and allows the system to work on repairing itself.

Working with Stretch and Properties of Skeletal Tissue

- Stretch- lengthen
  - The ability of a tissue to lengthen (stretch) without damage
- Contractility- shorten or attempt to shorten
  - The ability of a tissue to shorten; this is unique to muscle tissue

- Elasticity- return to shape
  - The ability of a tissue to return to its former shape after it has been stretched
- Tensegrity- withstand pull
  - The ability of tissue to withstand a pulling force without damage
- Plasticity- mold and hold shape
  - The tissues ability to have its shape molded or altered and will hold shape; this is unique to connective tissue
- Weight bearing- compression
  - The ability of a tissue to bear a compressive force or weight from above it without damage
- Creep- pressure and time (yin, hatha, long holds etc.)
  - The gradual shape change of tissue from a sustained and applied pressure
  - This can be positive in the case of massage therapies or long-held yoga postures or negative in the cases of poor posture (ex: slouching at a desk all day leading to a tissue shape change in the upper back and chest)
- Thixotropy- heat (vinyasa, Hot 26, etc.)
  - The ability of a tissue to change from a more rigid gel state to a softer "sol" state allowing for more freedom in movement and for greater ability of circulation

Types of Stretch

Below we have listed some stretching vocabulary and techniques. There are many "methods" and "brands" of stretching which often misuse the scientific terminology. Many of the techniques out there such as yin yoga and PNF (Proprioceptive Neuromuscular Facilitation) simply use a particular pattern of these four elements of stretch. As we use different combinations of stretch we can see how this may be reflected on our many different styles of yoga.

Static Stretching

Static stretching means a stretch is held in a challenging but comfortable position for a period of time, usually somewhere between 10 to 30 seconds. In the case of static yoga stretches they may be held from 30 second up to 2 minutes or more. Static stretching is considered safe and effective for improving overall flexibility. However, we may consider that static stretching may be much less beneficial than dynamic stretching for improving range of motion for functional movement, including sports and daily activities.

Dynamic Stretching

Dynamic stretching means a stretch is performed by moving through a challenging but comfortable range of motion repeatedly, usually 10 to 12 times. Although dynamic stretching might feel more challenging to some students as it requires more coordination than static stretching (because of the movement involved). Note that dynamic stretching should not be confused with bouncing or ballistic stretching. Dynamic stretching is controlled, smooth, and deliberate, whereas bouncing stretching is uncontrolled, erratic, and jerky. The risks that may occur in a bouncing stretch far outweigh the rewards. Controlled movements lend stability and therefore decrease the chance of injury.

Passive Stretching

Passive stretching means you are using some sort of outside assistance such as body weight, a strap, leverage, gravity, another person, or a stretching device to help you achieve a stretch. With passive stretching, you relax the muscle you are trying to stretch and rely on the external force to hold you in place. Effort in a passive stretch should be minimal. Please use caution as there is always the risk that the external force will be stronger than your flexibility, which could cause injury.

*Note: as an instructor this is where we must be careful when giving students hands on assists.

Active Stretching

Active stretching means you are stretching a muscle by consciously contracting the muscle in opposition to the one you are stretching without the use your body weight, a strap, leverage, gravity, another person, or a stretching device. With active stretching, you relax the muscle you are trying to stretch and rely on the opposing muscle to initiate the stretch or you are working with an eccentric contraction where the muscle is trying to contract as it is lengthening. Active stretching can be challenging because of the muscular force required to generate the stretch but is generally considered lower risk because you are controlling the stretch force with your own strength rather than an external force.

Breathing, Pranayama & Restorative Yoga

For the most part our breathing is automatic, however, we can regulate the manner, rate and force with which we breathe. Breathing is the manner in which oxygen is delivered into the body and CO_2 is removed from the body. The oxygen pathway mainly involves two major systems of the body: the respiratory system and the cardiopulmonary system.

Yogi Gupta says, "The mouth is for eating and the nose is for breathing." In yoga breathing is done primarily through the nose due to the warming properties of the sinus cavities that help both eliminate environmental offenders and heat the cool air before it hits the lungs. This creates *tapas*, a deep internal heat. Remember that the inhale is stimulating while the exhale is relaxing. (With the exception of some intentional and rigorous pranayamas.)

Pranayama and Restorative Yoga

Breathing is an internal system that operates automatically yet can also be consciously controlled. Awareness of every inhalation and exhalation is not the goal of yogic breath training, rather awareness is used as a tool of training the breath. The goal is to shape automatic breathing so that it flows optimally—in a deep, smooth, and effortless rhythm. Training also helps bring the various influences on breathing to conscious awareness. And it makes breathing strong enough to resist the disruption of harmful influences: stress, pain, and negative emotions.

As we know, when we connect to the breath we notice a shift from our outside world to our internal self and the arrows of attention draw inward. This is true in any yoga practice. Invite students to become the witness of their breath and thoughts without judgment. Remind students that if the mind wanders, to come back to the breath and not get discouraged. Eventually, this will become second nature. We learn by repetition.

The beginning of class or in between postures is a wonderful time to add pranayama exercises such as *nadi shodhana* or *dirga pranayama*. These practices help to relax and focus the mind and body and can be a wonderful tool for any student struggling with the monkey mind.

Try combining *nadi shodhana* with *ujjayi* for 3-7 minutes encouraging students to explore how long they can extend the length of the inhale and exhale. Counting the length inhales and exhales is another tool to help focus the mind on the breath.

Nadi Shodhana

Nadi shodhana is a purifying as well as a balancing pranayama. This practice of *nadi shodhana* purifies the network of energy channels in the body, and balance the coordination between right and left sides of the brain and right and left lungs.

To begin bring your right hand up to your nose. Gently block the right side of the nose with your thumb and inhale through the left nostril. Close off the left nostril with your right ring finger and then open the right nostril and exhale. Breathe in again through the right nostril then close it off with your thumb and open the left nostril to exhale. Alternate back and forth between the right and left nostrils.

Surya & *Chandra* Breathing: Sun/ Moon Breathing

The technique is the same and *Nadi Shodhana* except you will isolate one passageway and only follow one direction or channel. *Surya pranayama* begins the inhale through the right and each exhale is through the left. *Chandra pranayama* begins the inhale through the left nostril and each exhale is through the right nostril.

3 Part Breathing

Belly, thoracic and clavicular breathing is directed in sections to learn how to isolate the movement of the breath and train the accessory muscles of breathing. Begin breathing down into the base of the belly continue to fill the breath up into the ribs and sides of the body, then keep the same inhale going all the way to the top of the clavicles. As you exhale reverse the process and try to empty the air from the chest down to the ribs down to the base of the belly. Repeat for several rounds.

Ujayii: The Victorious Breath

Ujayii breathing is a form of pranayama that produces a soft and subtle sound by creating friction in the throat. It is a similar sensation to a "ha" sound or the way you would softly constrict your throat to try to fog up a mirror of pair of glasses before cleaning them. The inner throat is constricted by gently tightening the inner muscles at the glottis; the narrow opening forces the air to compress at a different rate and cultivates the friction needed to produce an internal heat. The external muscles of the throat should be relaxed. It is not a "Darth Vader" breath. *Ujayii* can be practiced with belly breathing or with the belly engaged.

Tips for breathing in a restorative yoga practice

- Move the belly with the breath. In some postures it may be helpful to place a sandbag or rolled blanket on the belly. Ask students to feel the weight on the belly and press the belly into the prop to deepen the breath.

- Allow the exhales to lengthen and pause at the bottom of the exhale. When we are stressed, the breath becomes short and high in the chest. Lengthening the breath creates a relaxation response within the entire body.

- Follow the breath all the way in and follow the breath all the way out.

- Breathe with the entire body. When we relax and slow down the rhythm of the breath, The body breathes like the waves of the ocean, uninterrupted by sharp movements. The exhales become twice as long as the inhales. Cue students to lengthen the exhale by 1 or 2 seconds deepening a sense of peace.

HTTP://tiny.cc/checkdr (Great article from the Mayo Clinic on when one should check with your doctor about physical exercise.)

General Precautions

All students come to the practice with a different story in their bodies. The crossroads of their many histories include but are not limited to a client's personal bone structure, past injuries, current level of fitness, and emotional state. We will all need to adjust for our bodies unique nature. That said some injuries or pathologies need more attention than others. Yoga should compliment our medical treatments, it is NOT a replacement for medical advice.

Spine:

- Degree and severity of injuries vary greatly. Some individuals have conditions such as herniations, bulging discs or spinal stenosis with no pain at all; while others have extreme pain sensations.

- No compression or pressure should be placed directly on an acutely injured area.

Joint Replacements:

- Knees: NO Virasana (Hero's Pose) or Balasana (Child's Pose). Refrain from extreme flexion of the knee, especially with the addition of weight bearing.

- Hips: NO Virasana (Hero's Pose). Refrain from extreme internal rotation of the femur as this can cause a dislocation of the bone from the hip socket. Avoid Lotus Pose and Lotus variations. Use caution with regards to deeper flexion and extension of the leg.

Hernias:

- Abdominal: Avoid pressure on the abdomen

- Groin: Avoid deeper stretches such as Bhekasana Variation (Frog Pose) and Upavistha Konasana (Wide Angle Seated Forward Bend). Refrain from deeper hip flexion and core work.

Headaches:

- Props such as a loose head wrap can be used or blocks to place under the forehead (Child's Pose, Down Dog) or top of the head (Uttanasana); avoid inversions.

Pregnancy:

- Not recommended for women over 20 weeks pregnant to lay horizontal on their backs (use inclines). Use caution with twists. NO *kapalabhati*, *bhastrika*, or *nauli* breathing.

44

Section 3

Asana (Postures)

"There is deep wisdom within our flesh, if we can only come to our senses and use it." -**Elizabeth A. Behnke**

Props

Use your imagination and the possibilities for support are endless.

Blankets

Wool army blankets or Mexican-style blankets will work nicely. Wool blankets are more firm than other blankets and hold their shape better in postures.

Blocks

Blocks are typically made out of a sturdy foam, cork or wood.

Bolsters

Bolsters are long, firm cushions. They come in many different shapes and sizes. Some are more round and others rectangular.

Yoga Mat

Use any standard yoga sticky mat.

Note: an extra mat besides the foundation mat is very helpful to support insteps, ankles, spine, etc. depending upon the posture.

Straps

6-9 foot straps are used to extend reach. Buckles come in D-rings and quick release. Quick release are easier to get into and out of. D-rings are often more durable.

Sand Bags

These bags are filled with sand to provide additional pressure and weight to the posture.

Eye Pillow

Eye pillows are filled with flax or rice. They come scented and unscented. Eye pillows keep out the light. Be cautious in instructing as too much pressure can be injurious to the corneas. Use a covering that can be removed and washed or disposed of for hygienic purposes.

Folding Chair

Use a standard metal folding chair.

Blanket Folding 101

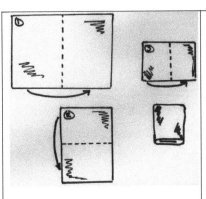	**Standard Fold** Fold an open blanket in half three times from short end to short end. Be sure to keep the folds smooth and avoid lumps.
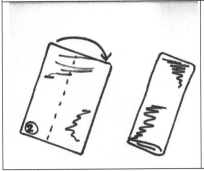	**Single Fold** Begin with a standard fold, then fold in half once more from long end to long end. Even folds now create more comfort later.

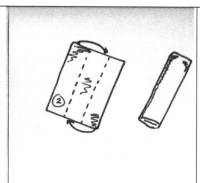	Double Fold Begin with a standard fold, then fold the blanket in thirds. The outside edges fold toward the mid-line from long end to long end. *I like to store my wool blankets this way, since it is the fold I use most often.*
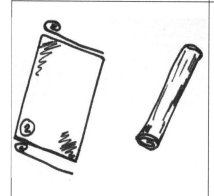	Standard Long Roll Begin with a standard fold, then roll the blanket tightly from long end to long end. This makes a perfect pranayama roll.

Asana Basics

- Give options to suit the unique needs of each student, then allow for all to rest in a neutral position.

- Skin should never rest on exposed carpet or floor; using a fully open blanket can prevent this.

- Cover students with a blanket to keep the heat in as necessary.

- Placing blankets be sure that it is smoothly rolled or folded; a blanket that is all balled up or uneven will make the body feel uneven and unsettled instead of the desired intention for support.

- Supine position for longer periods can be too much pressure and aggravate the low back .

Transitions

- Allow enough time for mindful transitions (3-4 minutes); this can include some time to lie on one side.

- If a pose is two-sided, invite the students to transition

slowly to the second side; no rush.

- Certain postures may require you to instruct the class to use minimal muscular effort; in some cases you and/or your assistants may need to offer more support to students through these transitions; be mindful in offering help to each student throughout your session.

- Backbending postures can be very vulnerable for students; have them roll to one side for a few breaths.

- A few rounds of cat/cow movement can be very nice after lying flat for longer periods.

- If both legs were bent in a posture, elongating them and stretching them out with awareness of the breath one leg at a time gets the blood flowing once again evenly in the extremities.

Vocal Cues

- Be clear! Specific direction is very important. Remember restorative yoga is the receptive side of yoga and requires a different energy. (Note: that does not mean whispering or inauthentic soft yoga-speak. Students still need to hear you. "Gentle" does not mean seductive speaking).

- Remind students that the props may have to be shifted until maximum release can be achieved encourage them to take steps necessary to get more comfortable. Let them know it is OK to call you over for assistance.

Useful Cues and Phrases:

Phrases and vocal cues are endless. Be creative, but be mindful not to over talk or rattle your cues off rather let them come naturally. Try ahead of time to get comfortable with your verbiage.

Be authentic. Do not parrot phrases just because it sounded good when someone else said it. Use what truly resonates with you and speak from the heart.

Get a thesaurus! Slowly and gently are the 2 most overused words in restorative yoga. Expand your vocabulary to create variety and texture to the fabric of your dialog with the class.

It is nice in each pose to indicate the benefits without over explaining. (EX: "twisting is good for elimination and keeping the spine supple.) You do not have to list a benefit for every posture. Too much information can sound robotic or like you are following a checklist. Our role as an educator is to create a safe space for others to have and enjoy their own experience. Strive to create an atmosphere that seems effortless to the students.

List some of your favorite guiding imagery phrases:

_____

_____

_____

_____

_____

_____

_____

_____

_____

_____

_____

_____

_____

_____

_____

_____

_____

Asana Types & Considerations

FORWARD BENDS:

(spinal flexion coupled with hip flexion or anterior tilt of the pelvis) expose the yang side of the body (the back side or posterior chain) and hold the yin side of the physical form (the front side or anterior chain) in a space that is calming and quieting. They place the body and mind toward the relaxation response. Forward bends can be followed by twists that are replenishing or back bends for opening and expansion.

BACK BENDS:

(spinal extension often coupled with hip extension and/or posterior tilt of the pelvis) lift the energetic system as they open the front of the chest (heart-center) and create room for the expansion of the lungs. Generally, they uplift energy and mood. Back bends can be followed by twists that are replenishing or forward folds for calming.

INVERTED POSTURES:

(Standing forward fold, headstand, downward facing dog) can invigorate the body and encourage productive and necessary circulation of the blood and lymph.

TWISTS:

(Spinal rotation and outer hip lengthening) are wonderful spinal balancers. Twists are often noted for the compressive squeeze and soak that stimulates the internal organs.

SAVASANA:

(corpse pose AKA final relaxation pose) is a neutralizing posture and often used to complete the practice. Note: Students with low back issues may find this pose uncomfortable if left in it for longer periods of time or may need additional support to remain in the pose. Crocodile (Prone Pose on the belly) can be a different option or seated meditation may be more supportive in certain instances.

Notes:

- *Try to keep your verbal cues fresh and pertinent. It is easy to go on autopilot.*

- *Find the most natural ways to encourage "letting go."*

- *Leave enough time for savasana and do not shortchange your students from fully experiencing a solid 10-20 minute relaxation.*

- *Watch for such as an arm suspended in the air, space behind the knees or the neck.*

- *Offer as much support as possible in any restorative posture.*

- *The more comfortable a student becomes, the deeper they can slip into release.*

Prone Pose

(Surfer Pose)

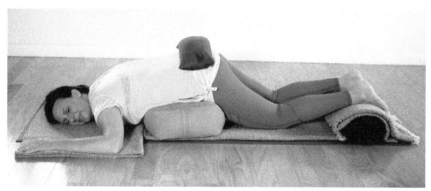

ASANA TYPE: FORWARD BEND & BACK BEND

Props Needed:

- One bolster
- Two or more blankets

Optional

- One sandbag

How To:

1. Set the bolster midway on the mat with a rolled blanket toward the base of the mat, begin in a tabletop position placing the hips over the bolster and ankles over blanket.

2. Lower the body down, allowing the hips to lay over the bolster.

3. Lower the torso onto the earth, and take the arms out to the side in the shape of a goal post.

4. Switch the direction of the head halfway through your hold time, hands may tuck under the supports or rest at your side.

Relax here for 2-20 minutes.

Benefits:	Cautions:
• Relieves stress and fatigue • Stretches low back • Relieves back and neck pain when properly supported	• Diarrhea • Pregnancy

Tips/Variations:

- Breathe fully: Feel an expansion of the back ribs with each inhalation.

- Place a sandbag on the sacrum.

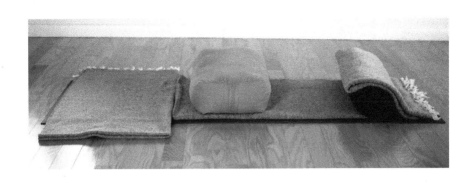

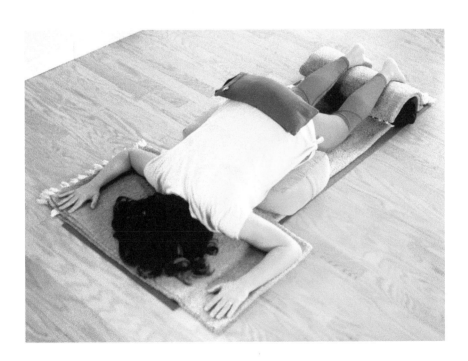

61

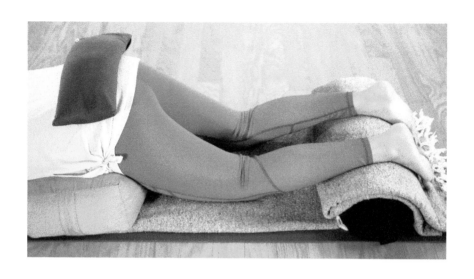

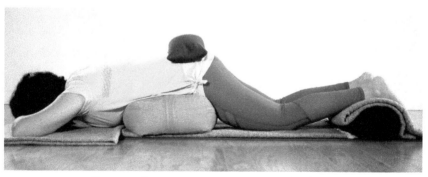

Optionally, arms can support the head

Child's Pose

(Balasana)

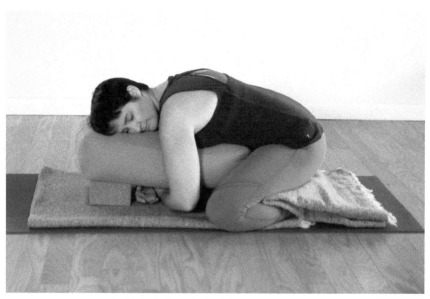

ASANA TYPE: FORWARD BEND

Props Needed:

- One bolster
- Two blocks
- One or more blankets

Optional:

- Rolled mat

How To:

1) Sit on the heels with knees separated and big toes touching (this is different from Bhekasana in which the feet are separated).

2) Place two blocks on the ground and a bolster on top of the blocks.

3) Lower the torso onto the bolster .

4) Switch the direction of the head halfway through the hold time, hands may tuck under the bolster.

Relax in pose for 2-20 minutes

Benefits:	Cautions:
• Stretches ankles, thighs and hips • Relieves back and neck pain when properly supported	• Diarrhea • Pregnancy: widen knees, support more under hips. • Knee injuries

Tips/Variations:

- Place a blanket between the thighs and the calves for more comfort.

- Place a blanket on mat under the ankles if they are lifted.

- Breathe fully: feel an expansion of the back ribs with each inhalation.

- Place a sandbag on the sacrum.

- Rolled mat can support the ankles

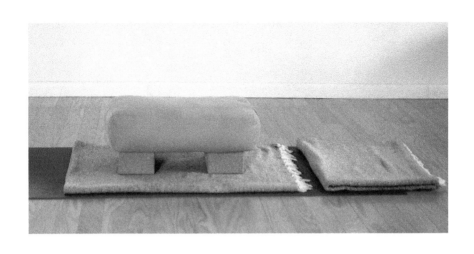

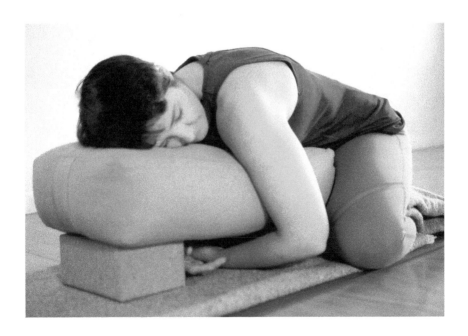

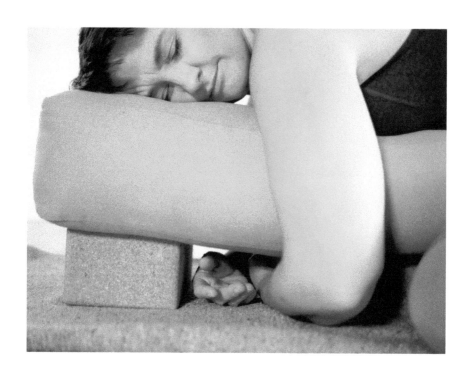

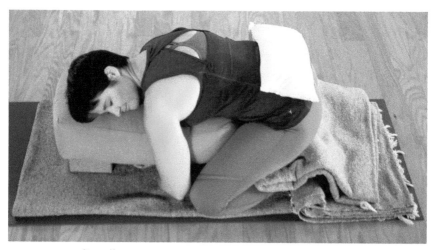

Sandbags can create a sense of grounding

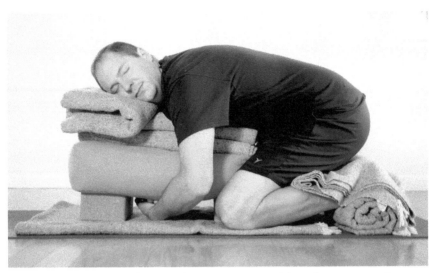

Blankets may be used to support ankles, hips or neck.

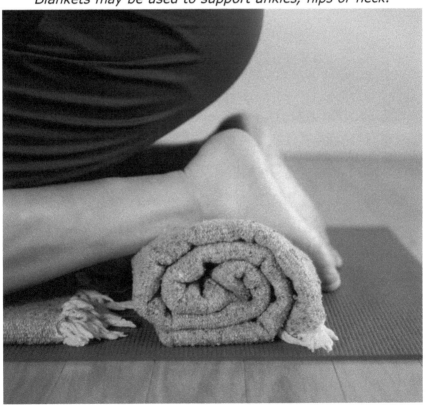

69

Frog Pose

(Bhekasana)

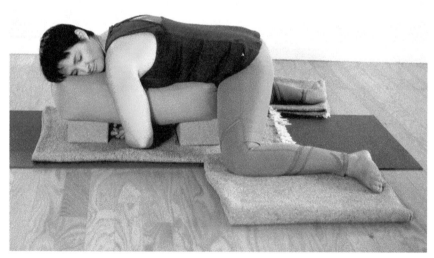

ASANA TYPE: FORWARD BEND

Props Needed:

- One bolster

- Two blocks

- Some blankets

Optional

- One sandbag

How To:

1. Place a bolster on top of 2 blocks.

2. Turn the feet out to the side and slide the knees away from each, keeping the feet in line with the knees (this is different from Balasana, when the feet are touching).

3. Lay on top of the bolster.

4. Switch the direction of the head halfway through

5. Hands may tuck under the blocks.

Relax here for 2-10 minutes.

Benefits:	Cautions:
• Relieves stress and fatigue • Stretches ankles, thighs and hips • Relieves Back and neck pain when properly supported	• Diarrhea • Pregnancy: widen knees, support more under hips. • Knee injuries

Tips/Variations:

- Build up height on top of the bolster with extra blankets if the groin area is tight.

- As needed, add extra blankets under the knees for comfort and cushion.

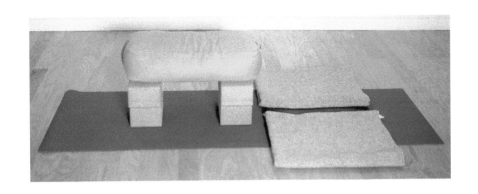

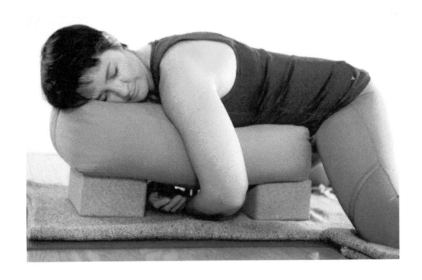

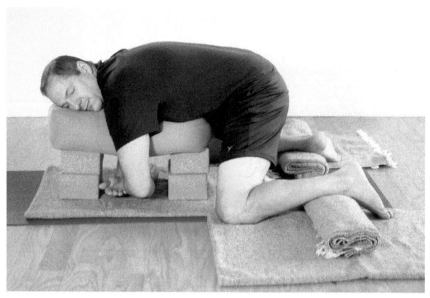

Additional props may be needed to add height

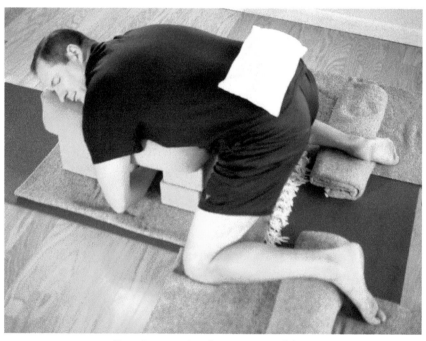

Passive assist from a sand bag

74

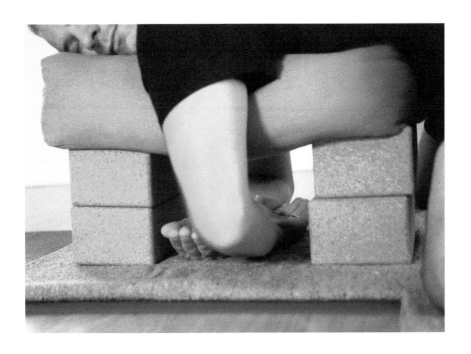

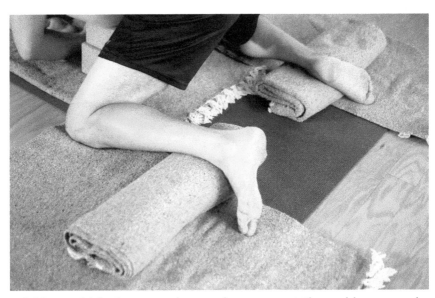

Additional blankets can be used to support the ankles or neck

75

Seated Forward Fold – Bolster Variation

Paschimottanasana

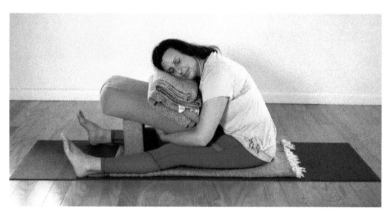

ASANA TYPE: FORWARD BEND

Props Needed:

- One block

- One bolster

- Two blankets

Optional:

- Extra mat or blanket

- Blocks to support forearms

How To:

1. Come to a seated position with the legs extended in front hip-distance, allow the toes to point up to the ceiling and make sure to sit on the sitting bones and not rolling onto the tail bone.

2. Place a block between the calves

3. Place a bolster over the thighs.

4. Settle the torso onto the cushion.

5. Rest the arms and hands alongside of the legs.

Relax here for 3-10 minutes

Benefits:	Cautions:
• Calms the mind	• Diarrhea
• Stretches the legs, muscles of the spine and the shoulders	• Use extreme caution with back injuries
• Compresses internal organs	

Tips/Variations:

- If the hamstrings are very tight, or there is a more limited range of motion, use the chair variation which is described next.

- Build up extra height to the bolster by adding blankets.

- A blanket may be added under the sitting bones to give lift to the hips.

- A rolled blanket under the knees can ease the hamstrings.

- Supporting the head with blocks or blankets may make the pose more comfortable for women with large breasts.

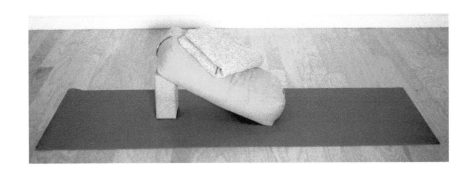

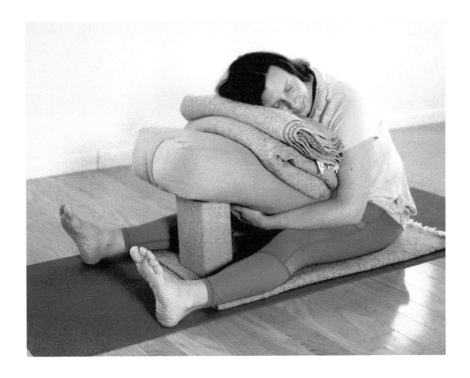

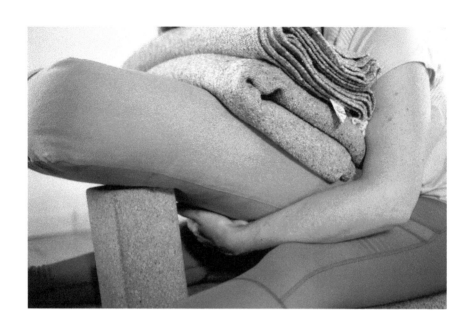

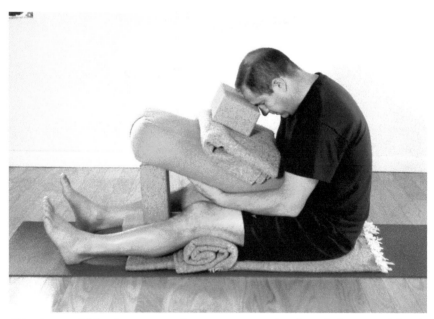

Blocks and blankets provide support to the head, legs and back

80

Seated Forward Fold – Chair Variation

Paschimottanasana

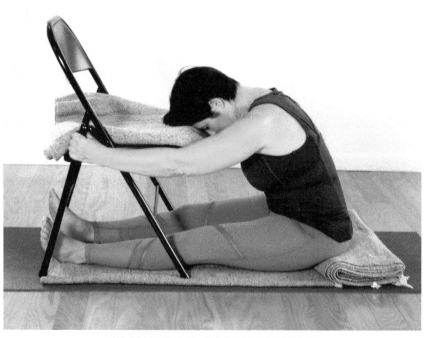

ASANA TYPE: FORWARD BEND

Props Needed:

- One folding chair
- Three blankets

Optional

- 4 blocks

How To:

1. Come to a seated position with the legs extended in front hip-distance, allow the toes to point up to the ceiling and make sure to sit on the sitting bones and not rolling onto the tail bone.

2. Slide the chair over the thighs with the back of the chair closest to the feet.

3. Reach the arms to the chair, and lay the upper body on the seat.

4. The arms may be crossed to make a wrist pillow and settle the forehead onto the back of the hands.

Relax here for 3-10 minutes

Benefits:	Cautions:
• Calms the mind	• Diarrhea
• Stretches the legs, muscles of the spine and the shoulders	• Pregnancy: Widen knees support more under hips.
• Compresses internal organs	• Knee injury

Tips/Variations:

- A blanket may be added under the sitting bones to give lift to the hips.

- Place blocks under the chair legs to lift entire chair up for people with tighter backs and hips.

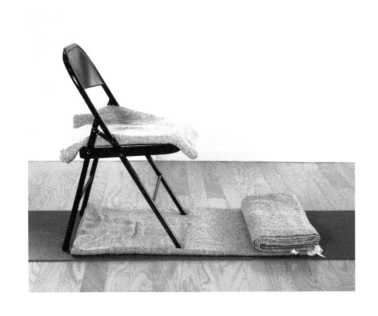

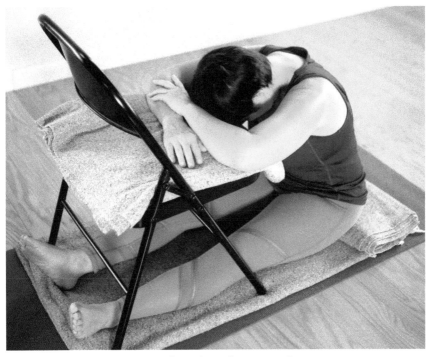

Arms may be placed across the seat

85

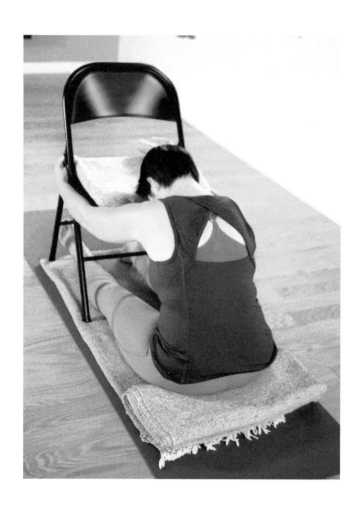

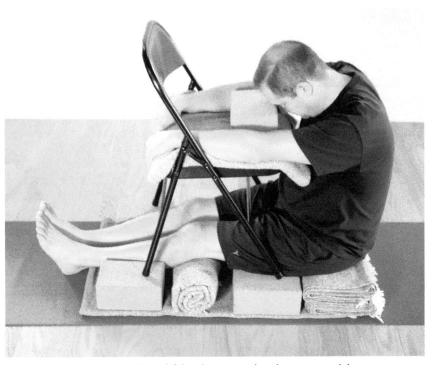

Chair raised and blankets under knees and hips

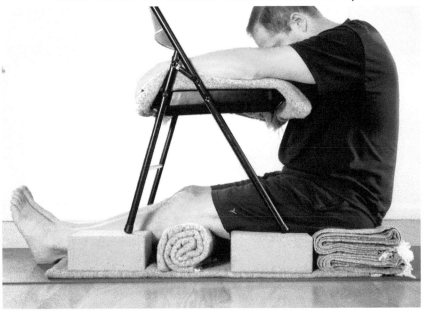

87

Supported Head-to-Knee

(Janu Sirsasana)

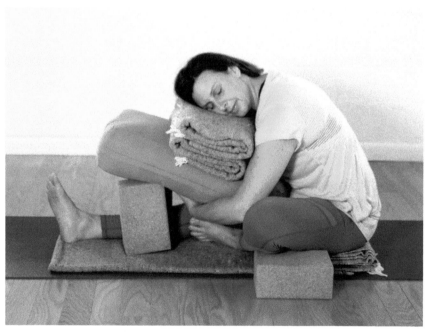

ASANA TYPE: FORWARD BEND

Props Needed:

- One bolster or chair

- Two blocks

- Blankets

How To:

1. Sit on the floor with the sitting bones propped on a folded blanket and the legs extended out in front, bend one knee and place the sole of that foot along the inner thigh of the other leg.

2. Place blocks on either side of the calf and place a bolster over the extended leg on the blocks.

3. Lengthen the torso over the bolster.

4. Allow your arms to rest along either side of the extended leg.

Relax here for 3-10 minutes. Switch sides and repeat.

Benefits:	Cautions:
• Stretches the spine, hamstrings and groins • Some find relief from menstrual discomfort and fatigue • Stimulates the liver and kidney meridians	• Diarrhea • Use caution with back injuries

Tips/Variations:

- If very tight or there is a more limited range of motion use a chair instead of a bolster.

- Increase height to the bolster by adding blankets or block.

- Add a blanket under the sitting bones to give lift to the hips.

- Use extra blocks to support the bent knee if the inner thigh is tight.

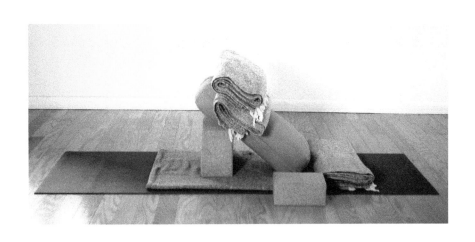

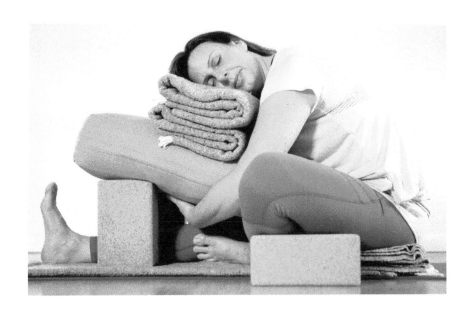

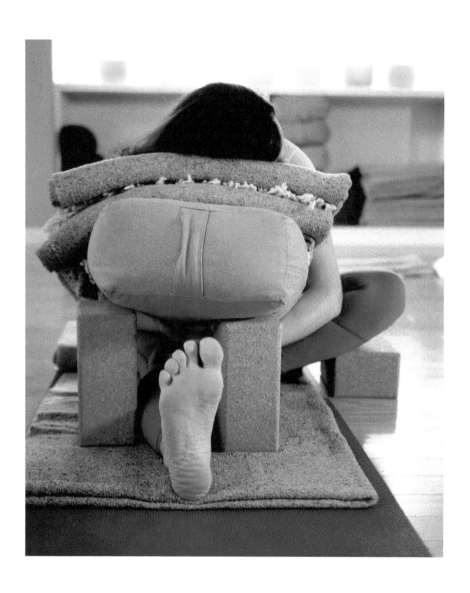

Half-Hero's Forward Fold

Triang Mukha Eka Pada Paschimottanasana

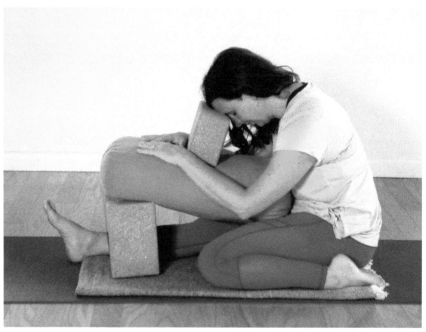

ASANA TYPE: FORWARD BEND

Props Needed:

- One blanket
- Three blocks
- One bolster

How To:

1. Sit on the floor with one leg extended out in front, bend the other knee and draw the heel alongside the hip.

2. Place blocks on either side of the calf of the extended leg.

3. Rest a bolster on the thigh of the extended leg and the blocks.

4. Lay the torso on the bolster, rest the arms along side, forehead may rest on the bolster, a folded blanket or a block.

Relax here for 3-10 minutes. Switch sides and repeat.

Benefits:	Cautions:
• Calms the mind	• Diarrhea
• Stretches the legs, muscles of the spine and the shoulders	• Use caution with back or knee injuries
• Compress internal organs	• Caution for students who have had hip replacements!

Tips/Variations:

- A blanket may be added under the sitting bones to give lift to the hips and create a more relaxed pelvis.

- Be sure that the extended leg is fully supported and there is no pressure in the back of the knee.

- Increasing the height of the bolster supports may be helpful.

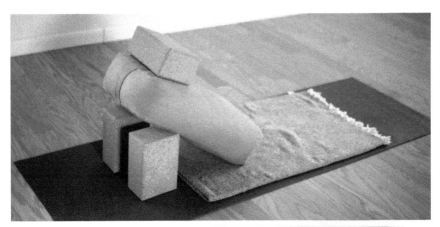

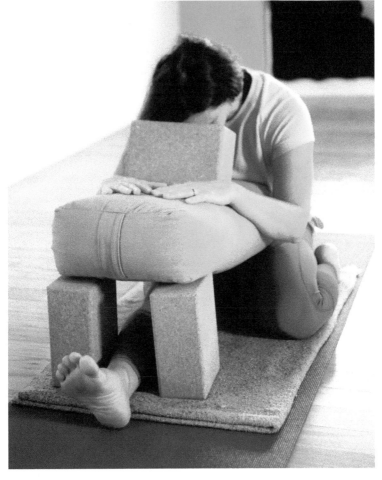

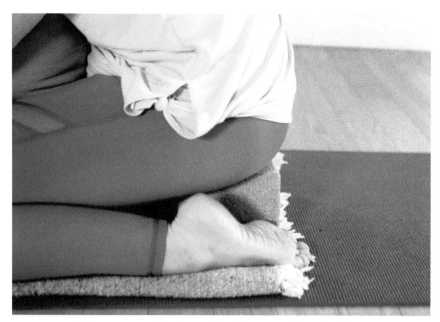

Sit up on a block or blanket to raise the hips

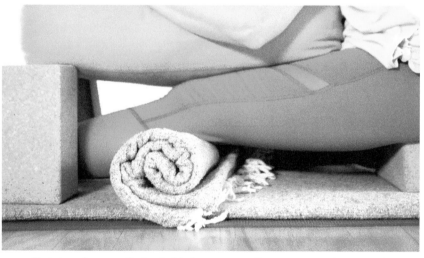

Raising knee of straight leg can relieve excessive strain

98

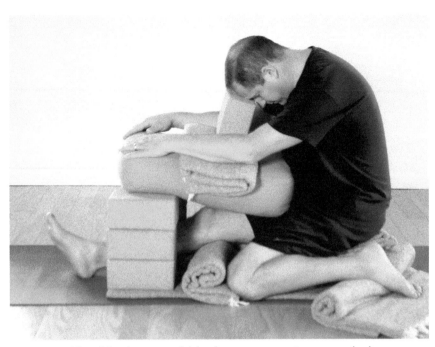

Use blankets and blocks to support as needed

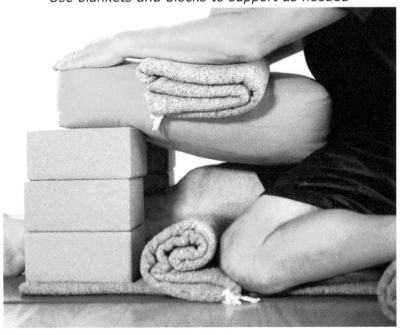

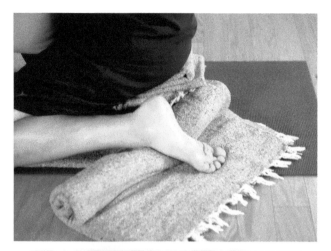

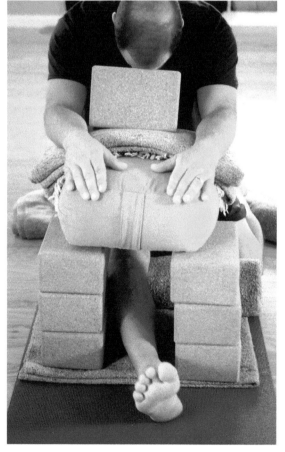

Supported Cow Face Pose

Gomukhasana

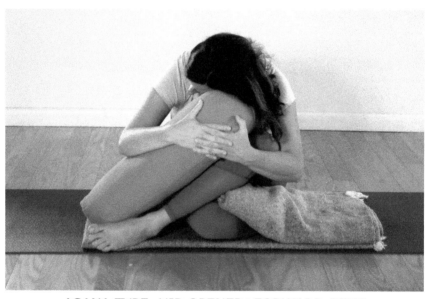

ASANA TYPE: HIP OPENER/ FORWARD BEND

Props Needed:

- One bolster

- Two blankets

How To:

1. Sit in dandasana, bend the knees placing the feet on the floor, slide one heel toward the other buttocks, cross the other leg over top, sliding the foot toward the hip.

2. Set a bolster on the top leg, fold forward and hug the bolster, rest forehead or cheek on the bolster.

Remain in the posture 1-3 minutes, switch sides and repeat

Benefits:	Cautions:
• Stretches the hips, thighs and gluteus muscles.	• Knee injury

Tips/Variations:

- Keep the bottom leg fully extended.
- Place a blanket between the knees if there is a large gap.

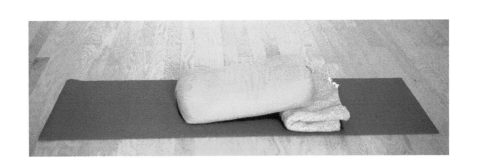

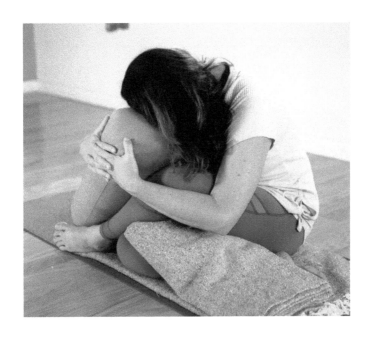

105

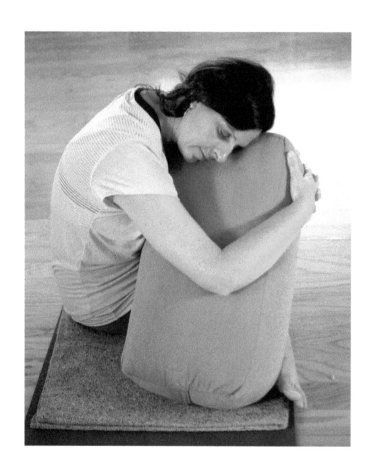

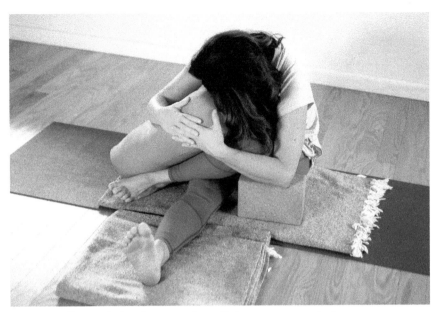

Extend the bottom leg if the pressure is intense

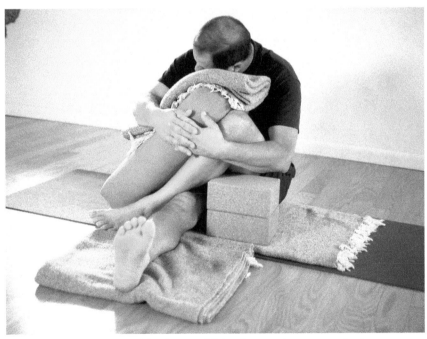

Use extra blocks and blankets where needed

107

Seated Wide Forward Fold

(Upavista Konasana)

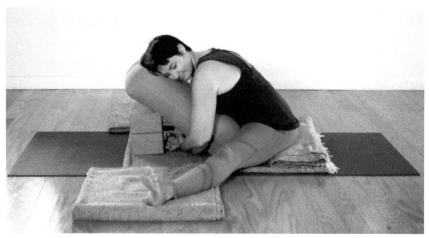

ASANA TYPE: FORWARD BEND

Props Needed:

- One bolster
- Two blocks
- Two blankets

How To:

1. Sit on the floor with sitting bones propped on a folded blanket and legs extended out wide legged in front.

2. Place a bolster between the extended legs, raise one end of the bolster with blocks.

3. Lengthen the torso over the bolster.

4. Allow the arms to rest along side or tuck them under the bolster.

Relax here for 3-10 minutes

Benefits:	Cautions:
• Stretches and releases the groins	• Low back injury
• Stretches the back of the legs	
• Calms the nervous system	

Tips/Variations:

- Use as many props as necessary to build up the height of the center pillar between the thighs for comfort in the low back and hamstrings.

- Blankets under the knees eases hamstring stretch.

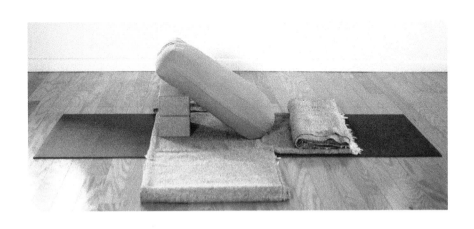

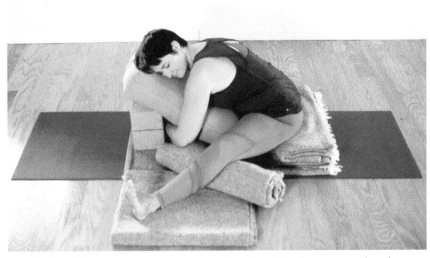

Rolled blankets may be placed under the knees and pelvis

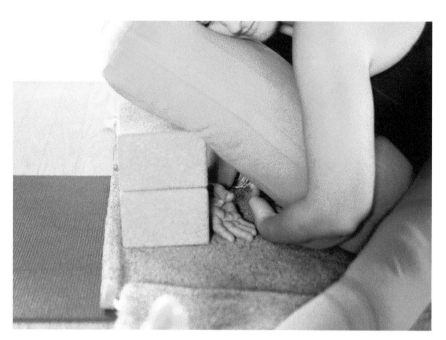

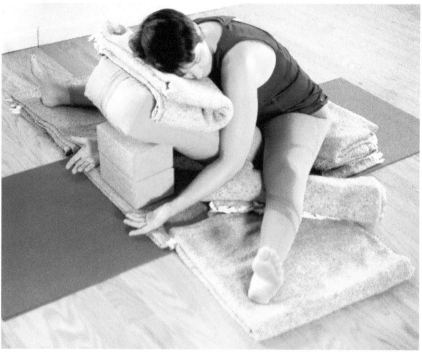

A folded blanket may be placed under the head

Sleeping Tortoise

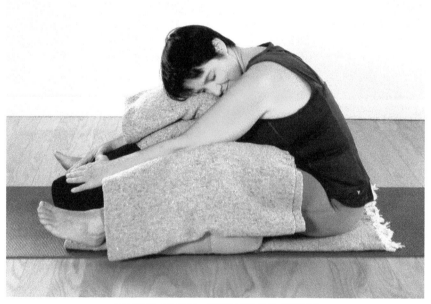

ASANA TYPE: FORWARD BEND

Props Needed:

- Three blankets
- Two bolsters

How To:

1. Place a bolster under the knees.

2. Lay the second bolster at the feet and the other end on the bolster under the knees.

3. Fold a blanket for the head on the bolster and place a blanket on each leg.

4. Hinge at the hips, folding forward. Lay the hands on the bolster. Lay the head on the folded blanket on top of the bolster.

5. Switch the direction of the head halfway through the hold time

Remain in the posture for 3-10 minutes

Benefits:	Cautions:
• Stretches and releases the groins • Stretches the back of the legs • Calms the nervous system	• Low back injury

Tips/Variations:

- A block can also be placed under the folded blanket for more propping.

- Add blanket under the sits bones to lift the hips, relax the pelvis and lumbar spine.

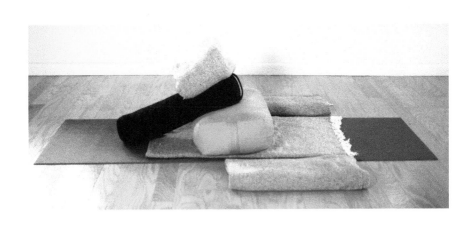

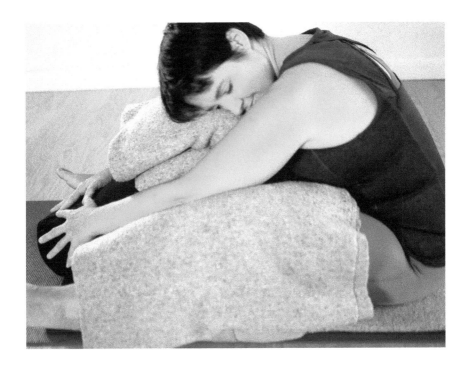

117

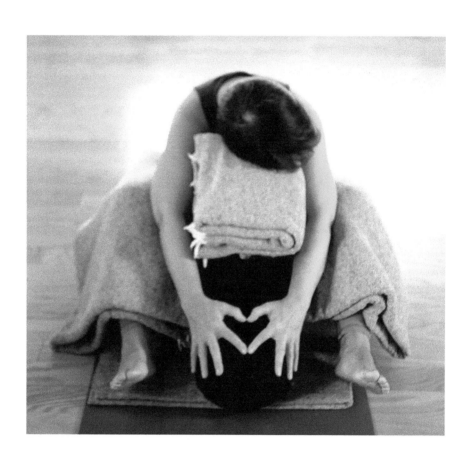

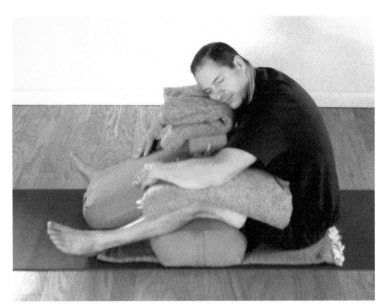

A larger bolster can be more supportive

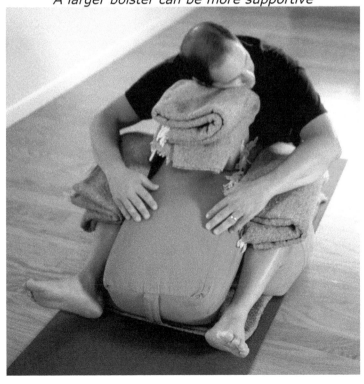

Hero Pose

(Virasana)

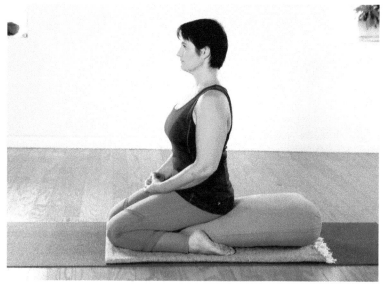

ASANA TYPE: SEATED

Props Needed:

- One bolster or a few blocks

- One or two blankets

How To:

1. Kneel on the floor (if needed, double up the mat or place a folded blanket underneath for extra cushion under the knees and shins) with the knees hip-distance.

2. Separate your feet wider than your hips.

3. Sit on a bolster or block .

4. Keep an anterior tilt to the pelvis and make an effort to sit upright, then relax within the effort.

Remain in the posture 3-30 minutes

Benefits:	Cautions:
• Stretches thighs, knees and ankles • Offers a steady position for pranayama and/or meditative practices	• Knee, ankle or foot injury

Tips/Variations:

- If the pose puts strain on the ankles, place a rolled blanket under them.

- Many find this pose challenging even with support and may not be appropriate for everyone.

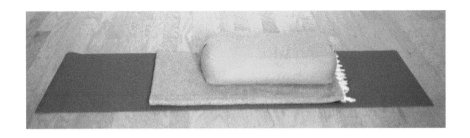

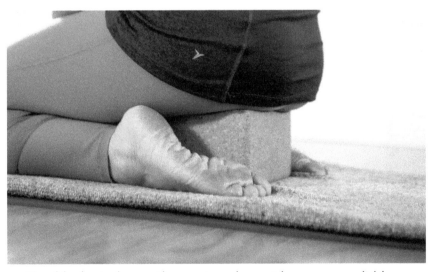

Use blocks to lower the seat and provide a more solid base

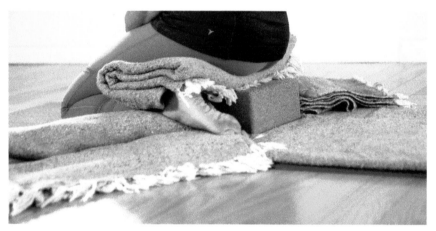

Blankets may support the ankle or raise the seat

Easy Seat

(Sukhasana)

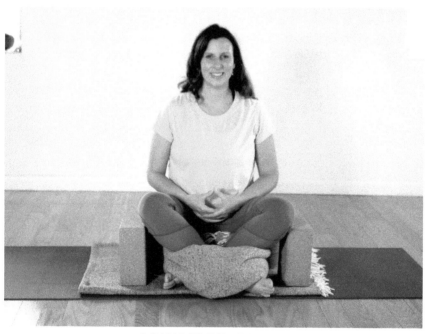

ASANA TYPE: SEATED

Props Needed:

- One bolster
- Two blocks
- Two blankets

Optional

- Strap

How To:

1. Sit on a bolster and place a second blanket rolled in the standard long roll, across the shin bones over top of the blanket.

2. Slide a block under each knee, keep an anterior tilt to the pelvis and make an effort to sit upright, then relax within the effort.

3. Place the hands on the lap or relaxed in a mudra (hand position).

Remain in the posture 3-30 minutes

Benefits:	Cautions:
<ul><li>Calms the brain</li><li>Strengthens the muscles of the back</li><li>Stretches the hips, knees and ankles</li></ul>	<ul><li>Knee injury</li><li>Coccyx pain</li></ul>

Tips/Variations:

- If the knees are higher than the hips, increase the height of the seat.

- This can be done leaning against a wall with the aid of a block between the wall and the shoulders.

- Placing a strap around the thighs can provide greater hip support.

- Sitting on a folded blanket will lower the seat.

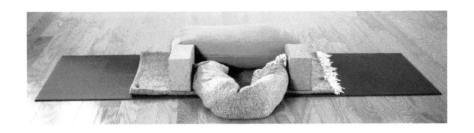

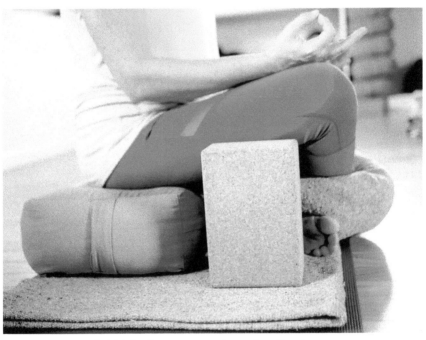

Add block to support under the knees

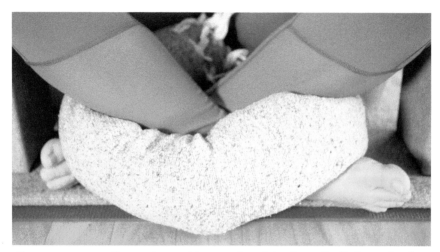

Ease pressure from the ankles with a blanket (Roll described at the beginning of the chapter)

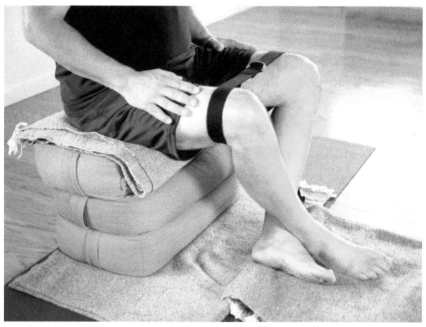

Chairs or extra bolsters can help support students with knee hip or spinal tension. Straps can stabilize the hips and knees

Easy Throne

(Easy Seat variation)

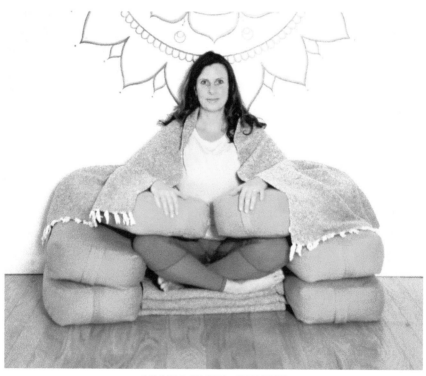

ASANA TYPE: SEATED

132

Props Needed:

- Six bolsters
- Many blankets

How To:

1. Stack blankets against a wall and place three bolsters on either side of stack.

2. Sit on blanket stack and draw top bolster over the knees

Remain in the posture 3-30 minutes

Benefits:	Cautions:
• Calms the brain	• Knee injury
• Stretches the hips, knees and ankles	• Coccyx pain

Tips/Variations:

- The deluxe version against the wall will have you feeling like royalty!

- Keep one blanket to wrap around like a shawl.

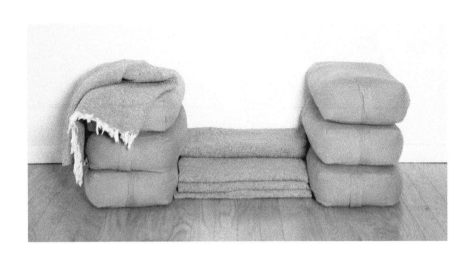

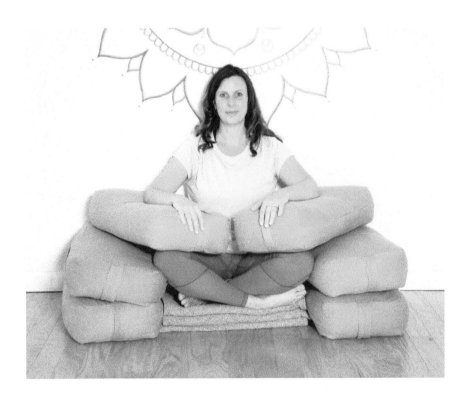

135

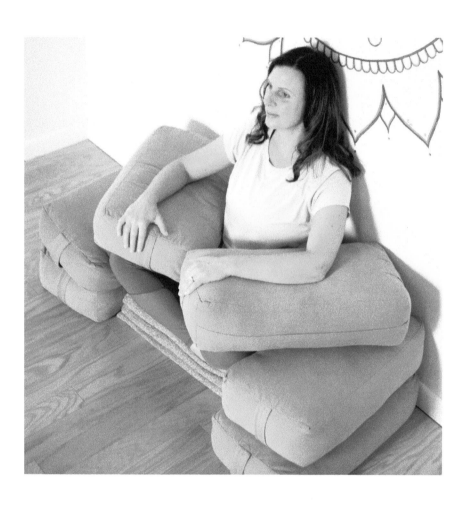

Fish Pose

(Matsyasana)

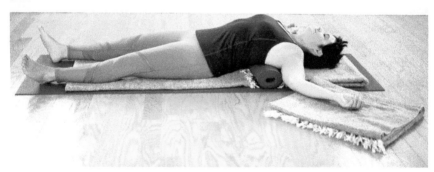

ASANA TYPE: BACK BEND

Props Needed:

- Three or four blankets
- An extra rolled mat

How To:

1. Lie in a supine position over rolled mat lined up crosswise under the shoulder blades.

2. Align the neck so that it is supported by the edge of the blanket and lay the arms out to the sides.

Remain in posture 1-5 minutes

Benefits:	Cautions:
• Opens the mid-back	• Migraines
• Lengthens the muscles of the belly	• Pregnancy (after 20 weeks)
• Improves posture	

Tips/Variations:

- Keep the muscles of the throat soft.

- Lay arms on the belly if shoulders are uncomfortable in the open position.

- For a more gentle backbend, try Mountain Brook Pose (next pose).

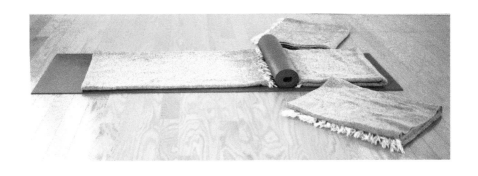

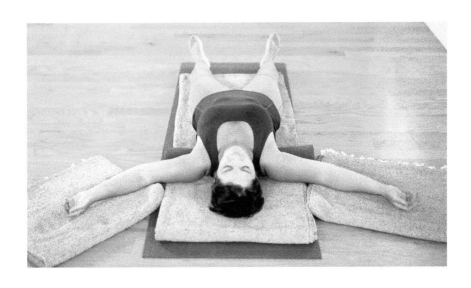

141

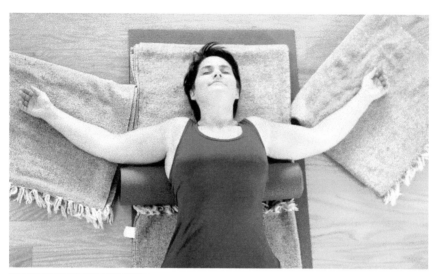

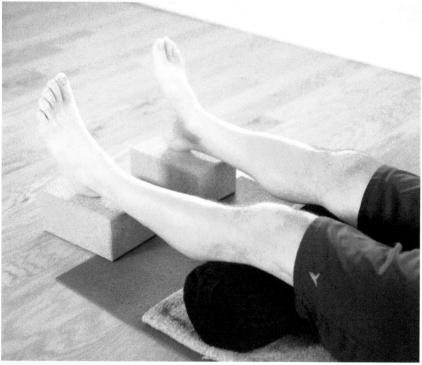

For low back sensitivity, support under the knees and lifting the feet will eases pressure in the knees

142

Mountain Brook Pose

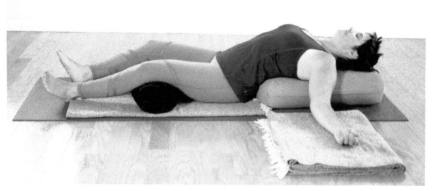

ASANA: BACKBEND & RELAXATION

Props Needed:

- Two bolsters
- One blanket

Optional

- One eye pillow

How To:

1. Place the short end of a bolster against the sacrum, lay over the bolster.

2. Slide a bolster under bent knees.

3. To release the posture, roll to your side into a fetal position then push up to a seated position.

Remain in the posture for 5-15 minutes

Benefits:	Cautions:
<ul><li>Opens chest and shoulders</li><li>Calms the body</li><li>Reduces fatigue</li></ul>	<ul><li>Back injury or discomfort</li></ul>

Tips/Variations:

- If the feet are in the air, place a blanket or blocks underneath the heels to support the ankles.

- Add a blanket under the neck for more cervical support.

- Place a sandbag across the belly just above the hips, noticing the rise and fall of the sandbag.

- Cover the eyes with an eye pillow and the body with a blanket.

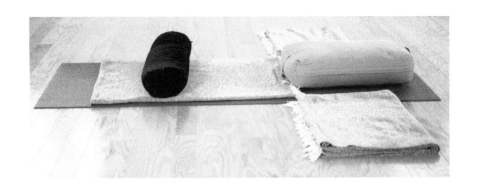

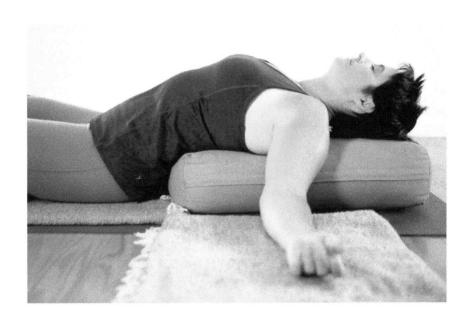

147

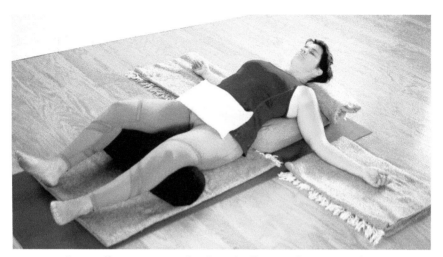

A sandbag across the low belly can be grounding

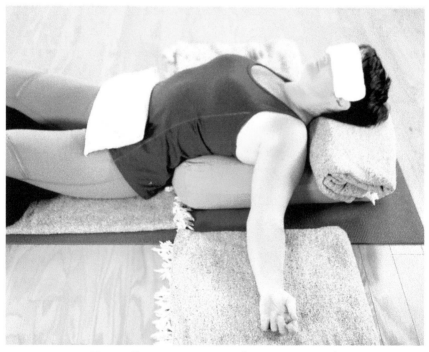

Eye pillows are a nice, luxurious touch

148

Pranayama Support

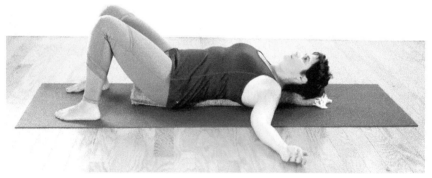

ASANA: BACKBEND

Props Needed:

- One rolled up yoga mat or blanket

How To:

1. Sit upright and place the end of the rolled up yoga mat against the sacrum.

2. Lie back, aligning the spine with the rolled up mat.

3. Open the arms and lay them on the ground to the side.

Remain in the posture for 3-10 minutes

Benefits:	Cautions:
• Opens chest and shoulders • Calms the body • Reduces fatigue	• Pregnancy over 20 weeks

Tips/Variations:

- For more support, use a rolled up blanket instead of a mat

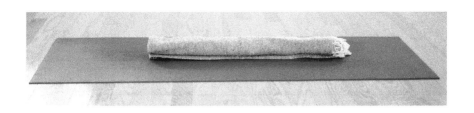

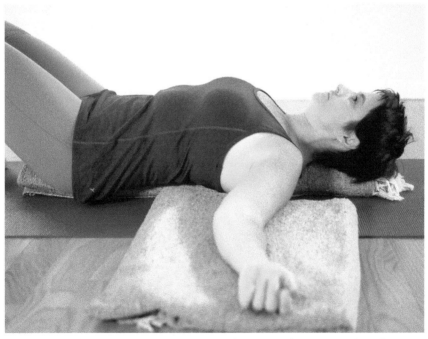

Raising the arms will decrease the stretch across the chest

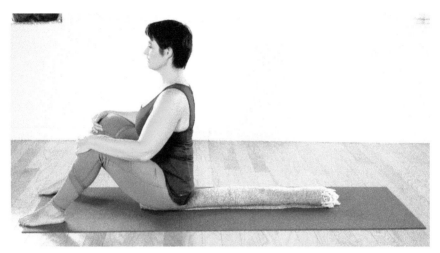

To enter the pose, sit against the base of the rolled blanket and curl back

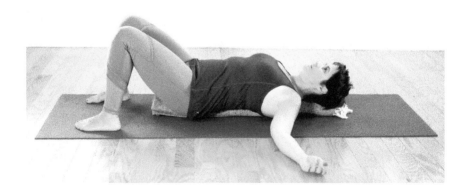

Reclining Bound Angle

(Supta Baddha Konasana)

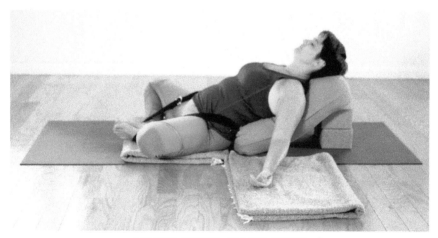

ASANA TYPE: BACK BEND

Props Needed:

- One bolster
- One strap
- Three blankets
- Four blocks

Optional

- One eye pillow

How To:

1. Sit in baddha konasana, make a strap into a loop and place it around the waist and the front of the feet.

2. Lie back onto a bolster running from sacrum-to-head and place a blanket under the head, blankets can be placed on either side under the arms for more cushion and support of the chest and shoulders .

3. Reach down to the strap and tighten the loop, blocks may be placed under the knees.

4. To release the posture loosen the strap and roll to one side, then push up to a seated position.

Remain in the posture for 5-15 minutes

Benefits:	Cautions:
• Opens chest and shoulders • Calms the body • Reduces fatigue • Stretches the hips and groins	• Knee injury • Groin injury

Tips/Variations:

- Do not tighten the strap until you are in the supine position or it can create discomfort.

- Keep the buckles of the strap resting in a way it will not dig into the skin.

- Adjustments can be made as the body settles into shape.

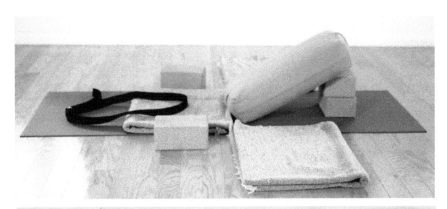

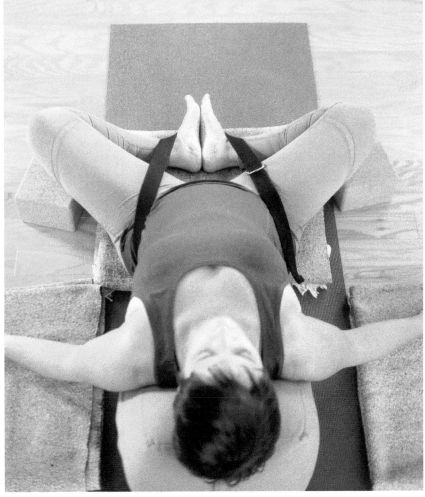

159

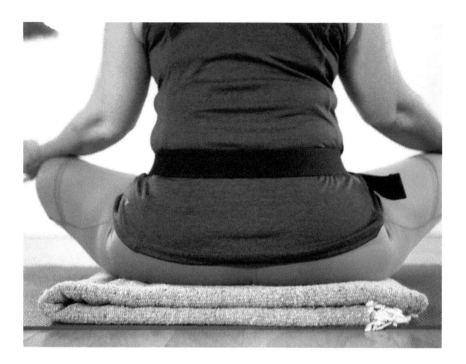

Strap Placement

The strap loop is placed at the top edge of the sacrum. Be careful not to let it slide into the low back. The front edge of the loop then hooks over the feet. Make sure the buckle is placed where it will not dig into the body. Wait until the body is fully reclined to tighten the strap. Tightening the strap too much, too soon will make it difficult to recline into the full pose.

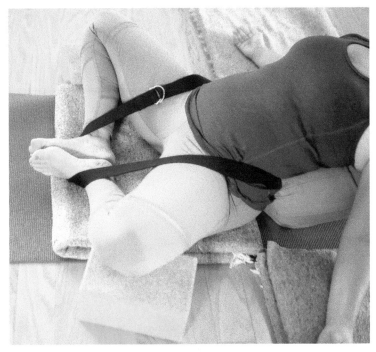

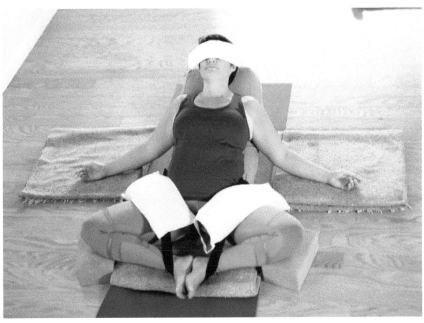

Sandbags and an eye pillow are lovely options

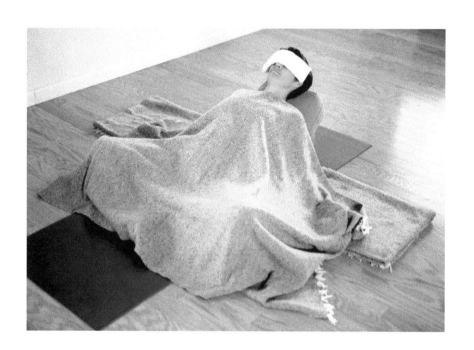

Bridge Pose

(Setu Bandha Sarvangasana)

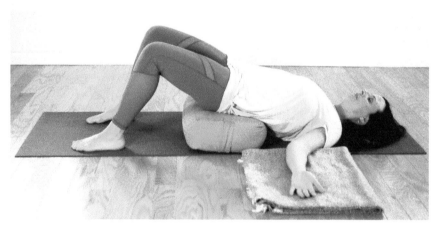

ASANA TYPE: BACK BEND

Props Needed:

- One bolster
- Two blankets

Optional

- Block

How To:

1. Lie on the back, bend the knees and place the feet on the floor hip-distance apart with heels close to the sitting bones.

2. Lift the hips up and slide a bolster underneath the sacrum (it may be necessary to move the bolster slightly forward or back to find the most comfortable resting place), lower the sacrum onto the bolster.

3. To release the pose lift the hips and slide the bolster out to the side, lower the hips back to the floor and roll onto the side.

Remain in the posture 1-5 minutes

Benefits:	Cautions:
• Stretches the shoulders, chest, spine and abdomen • Stimulates lungs • Opens the hip flexors	• Avoid this posture with injuries of the cervical spine

Tips/Variations:

- A strap just above the knees can support the legs.
- Different leg variations will direct opening to the hips flexors.
- Use a block to increase level of intensity.
- Keep the chin slightly lifted away from the chest so that the natural curvature of the neck is supported.

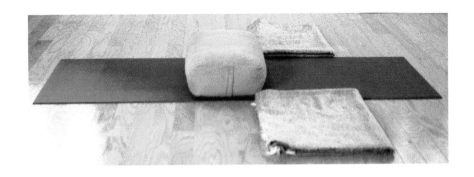

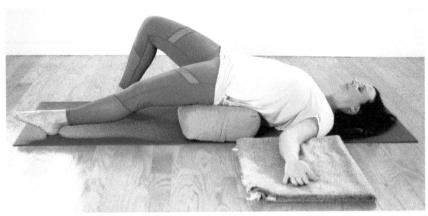

Alternate leg extensions will vary intensity and release

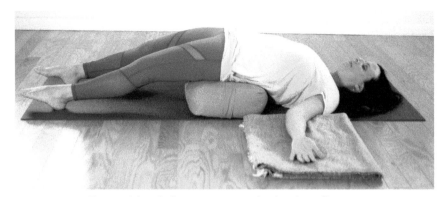

Extend both legs to stretch the hip flexors

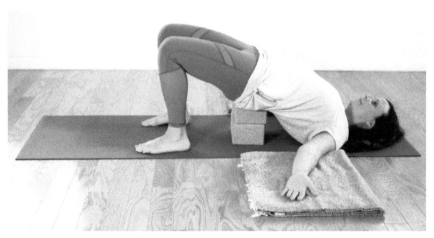

Use stacked blocks to increase backbend

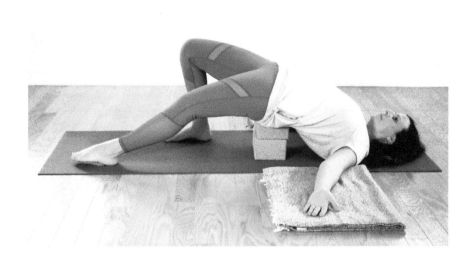

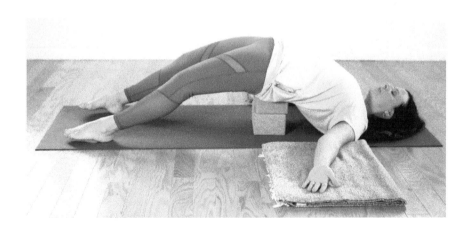

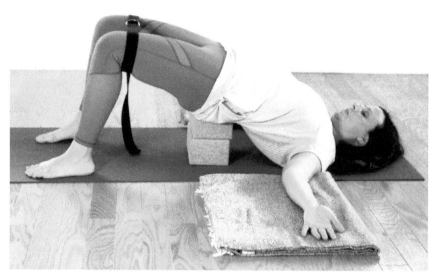

A strap can support the inner thighs

Half Moon Pose

(Crescent Posture)

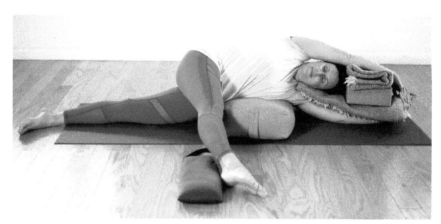

ASANA TYPE: LATERAL SIDE BEND

Props Needed:

- One bolster
- Two blankets
- One Sandbag

Optional

- One block

How To:

1. Lay over a bolster so that the lower ribs and waistline are supported.
2. Reach the arms overhead. Rest the head on the lower arm or additional blanket.
3. Draw the top leg forward, place above the sandbag and draw the bottom leg back.

Remain in the posture 1-5 minutes. Switch sides and repeat

Benefits:	Cautions:
• Stretches the obliques, intercostals and the latissimus dorsi muscles	• Rib cage injury • Shoulder injury

Tips/Variations

- Increase the stretch by drawing the top shoulder blade back in a diagonal opposition to the upper hip.

- Place a sandbag down the thigh and/or on the floor beneath the top foot to hold leg in place, the sandbag can then be moved up the floor to deepen the stretch of the top leg.

- If the shoulder doesn't feel comfortable, the top arm can be released in front of the chest.

- Use a block to support the top arm

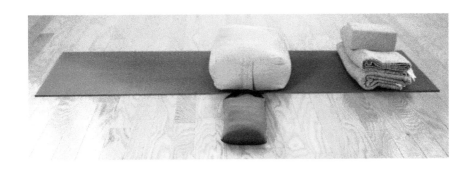

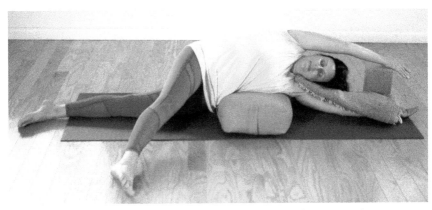

Sandbag can be removed to ease the stretch

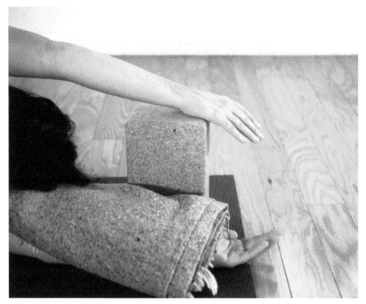

Vary hand position and support to change shoulder intensity

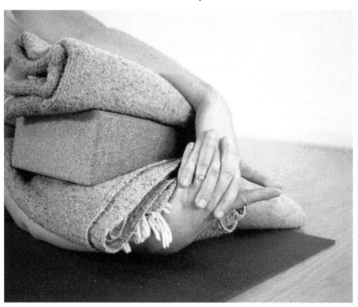

176

Side Lying to Twist

(Supine)

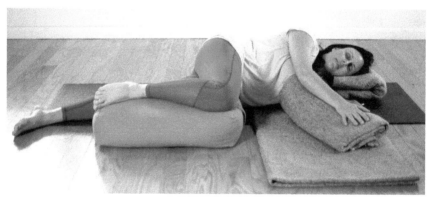

ASANA TYPE: TWIST

Props Needed:

- One bolster
- Three blankets

How To:

1. Lie on the side with a folded blanket under the head, place a bolster under the bent knee of the upper leg, pause and rest here for several breaths.

2. Reach the top arm back as the chest is rolled open into a twist, allow the arm to rest softly on the blanket behind.

Remain in the posture 1-5 minutes. Switch sides and repeat

Benefits:	Cautions:
• Stretches shoulders and hips	• Spinal injury
• Stimulates elimination	

Tips/Variations:

- Set the second blanket behind so that the twist can occur without disturbing the flow.

- If there is limited spinal rotation or tightness in the shoulders, the arm support may need to be elevated, do not let the back arm dangle in space.

- Knees and ankles should be fully supported.

- Side lying poses are great option for the prenatal population when lying on the belly is no longer appropriate or after 20 weeks at which time some pregnancies may experience vena cava syndrome when lying on the back.

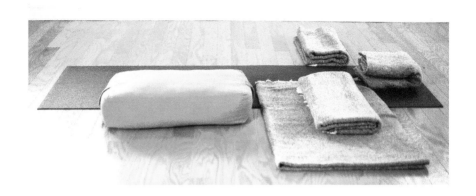

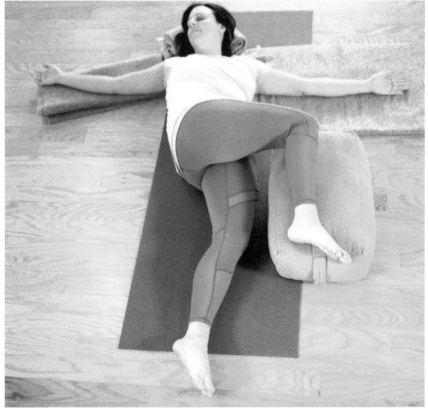

Open to full twist by reaching top arm behind

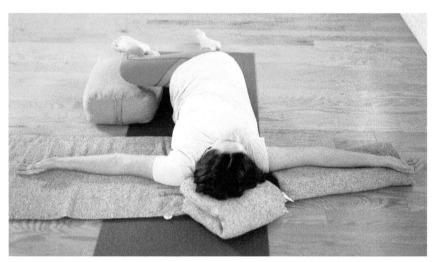

Raise the support of back arm to decrease intensity of the twist

Side Lying to Twist

(Prone)

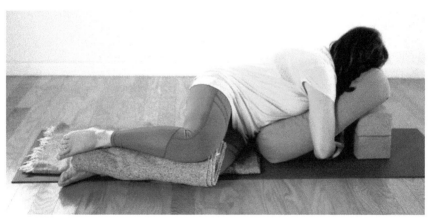

ASANA TYPE: TWIST

Props Needed:

- One bolster
- Two blankets
- Two blocks

How To:

1. Sit with one hip perpendicular to the bolster with legs in an L shape, place a blanket between the shins.

2. Turn the belly toward the bolster and lean into the support, arms can slide underneath the bolster.

Remain in the posture 1-5 minutes. Switch sides and repeat

Benefits:	Cautions:
• Stretches spinal muscles and hips • Stimulates elimination	• Spinal injury

Tips/Variations:

- For more neck stretch turn the head in the opposite direction of the knees, for less intensity turn the head in the same direction as the knees.

- Remove blocks under the bolster to reduce the angle.

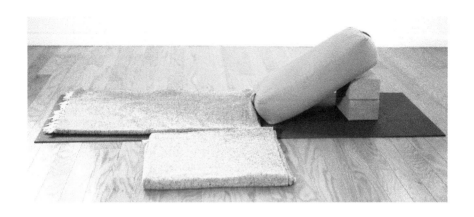

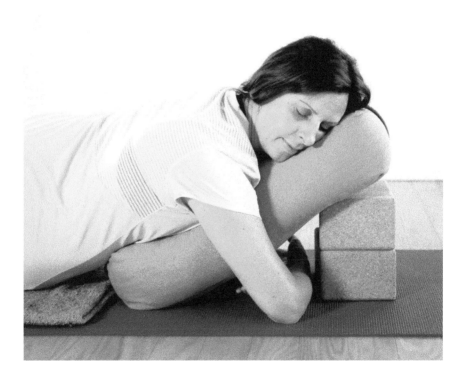

187

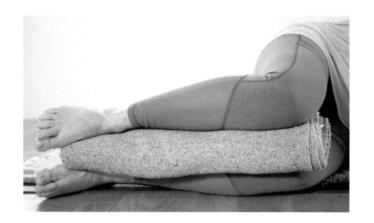

188

Pigeon Pose

(Eka Pada Kapotasana)

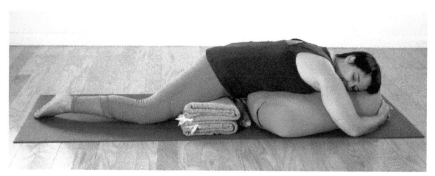

ASANA TYPE: HIP OPENER/FORWARD BEND

Props Needed:

- One bolster

- Two blankets

Optional

- One block

- One sandbag

How To:

1. Set a bolster at an angle. Place 2 stacked blankets across the mat, below the bolster.

2. Begin in tabletop position and slide a knee up to the outer edge of the front bolster, resting the back thigh and pelvis over the crosswise bolster.

3. Lower the torso over the front bolster and slide the arms under the space of incline.

Remain in the posture 1-5 minutes. Switch sides and repeat

Benefits:	Cautions:
• Opens the hip flexors and spine • Stretches the piriformis which can alleviate some sciatic nerve pain if the nerve is being stressed	• Knee issues

Tips/Variations:

- Elevate one end of the bolster with a block.

- Place a sandbag on the sacrum to ground the pelvis.

- If more height is needed additional blankets may be place over the front bolster.

- The bolster may be skipped, instead use a blanket for more stretch.

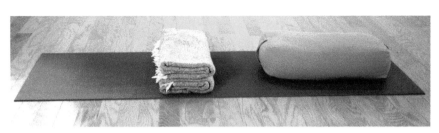

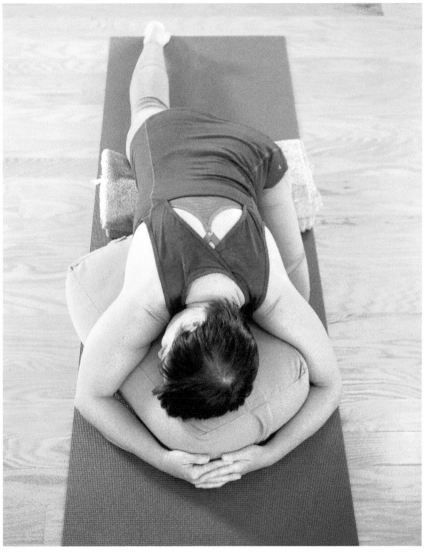

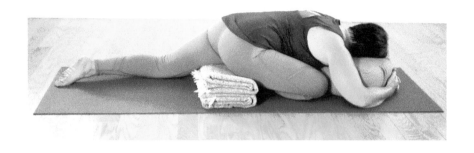

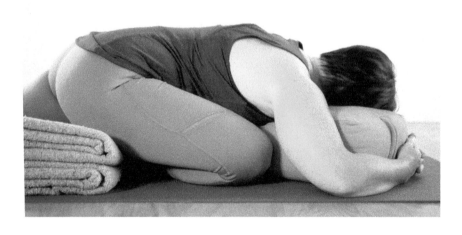

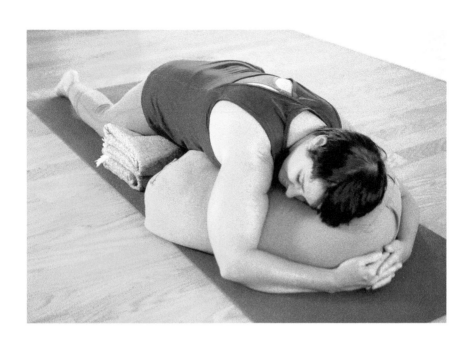

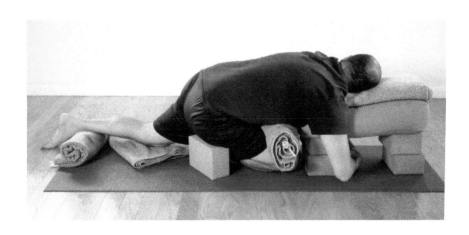

195

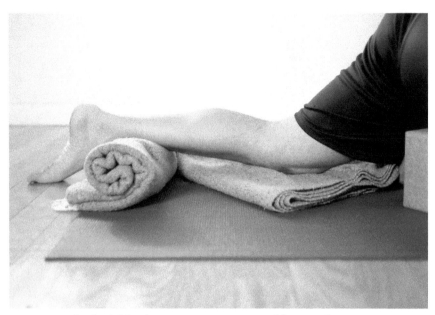

Rolled blankets can support ankles and torso

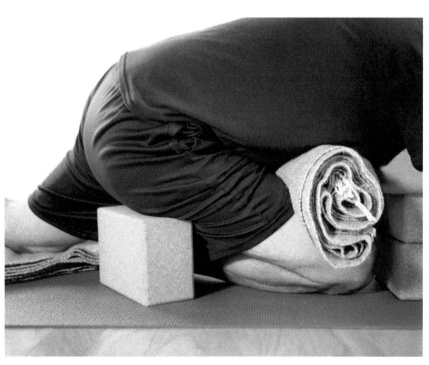

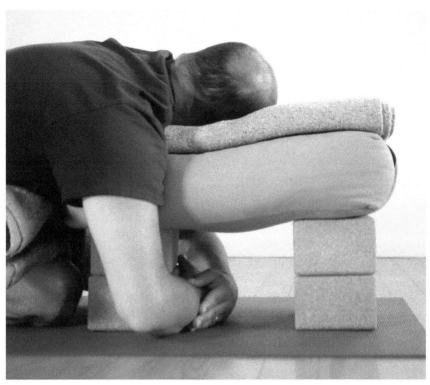

Use blocks to raise bolster and support the hips

Legs up the Wall

(Viparita Karani)

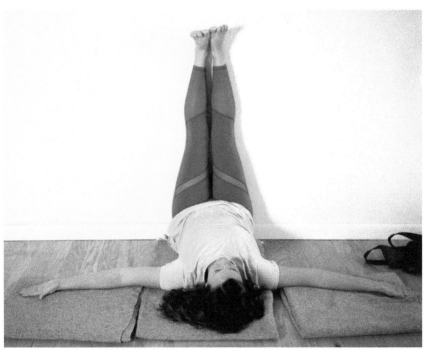

ASANA TYPE: INVERSION

Props Needed:

- Wall space
- Three blankets

Optional

- One bolster
- One eye pillow
- One strap
- One sandbag

How To:

1. Draw your legs up the wall (see photos for entry into pose).

2. Allow the weight of the legs to lean against the wall.

Remain in the posture 5-15 minutes

Benefits:	Cautions:
• Stretches the back of the legs • Relieves tired legs and feet	• Should be avoided with eye problems such as glaucoma • High blood pressure • Ear infections

Tips/Variations:

- Place a sandbag on the feet to ground the pelvis.

- Resting hips on top of a bolster, will decrease hamstring stretch and add a gentle backbend.

- Place a strap around the legs to hold them together.

- It can be a bit tricky to guide students onto the wall. See following images for visual guide.

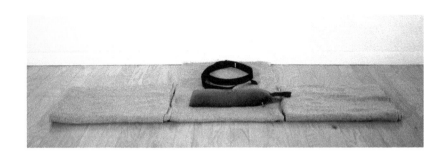

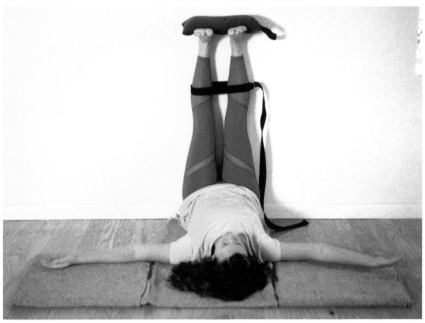

A strap can hold the thighs together in all of the variations. A sandbag placed on the feet can cultivate a feeling of grounding.

Entry for Viparita Karani:

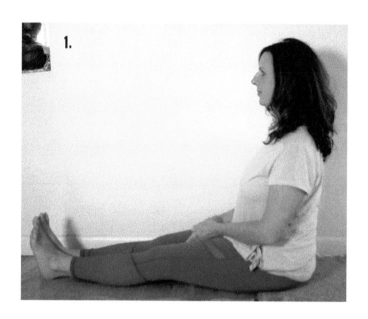

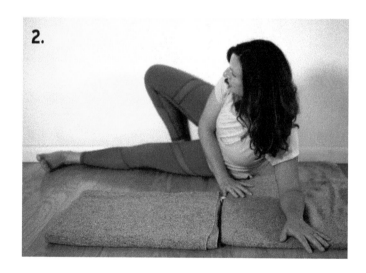

3.

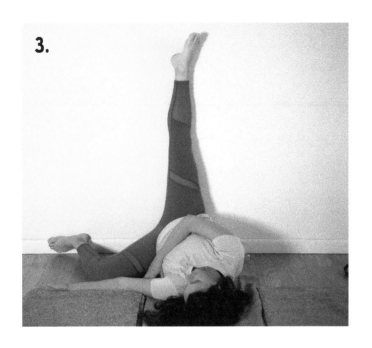

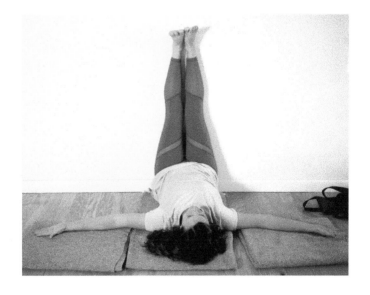

Bent-Knee Hip Opener

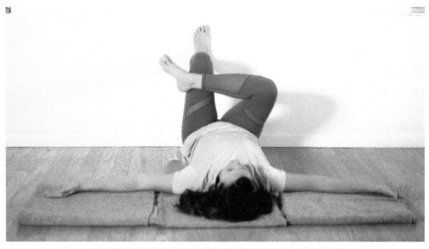

ASANA TYPE: INVERSION/HIP OPENER

Props Needed:

- Wall space

How To:

1. Begin in Viparita Karani (above), without the bolster.

2. Cross one leg over the other knee opening the crossed knee toward the wall in a figure 4 position.

3. Bend the straight leg and place the sole of the foot against the wall.

Remain in the posture 1-3 minutes. Switch sides and repeat

Benefits:	Cautions:
• Stretches the hips and groins	• Knee injury • High blood pressure

Tips/Variations:

- Slide the foot down the wall down to intensify the stretch or up the wall to decrease intensity.

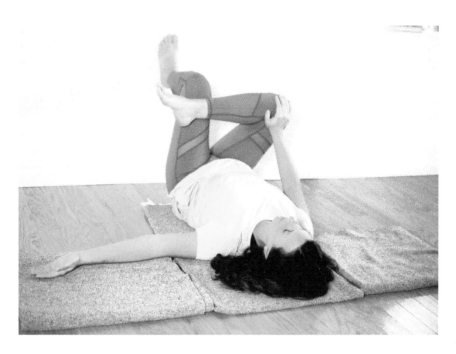

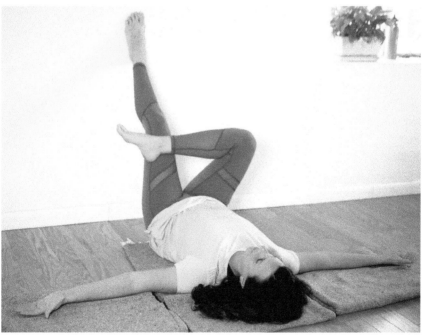

Straightening the leg decreases the stretch

Inverted Reclining Bound Angle

Supta Baddha Konasana Inversion

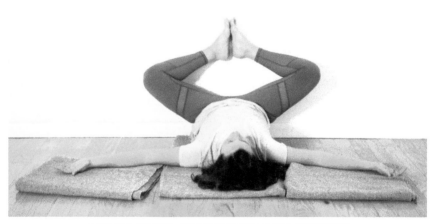

ASANA TYPE: INVERSION/HIP OPENER

Props Needed:

- Wall space

Optional

- Two blocks

How To:

1. Begin in Viparita Karani (above), without the bolster.

2. Bending the knees, bring the soles of the feet together and allow the knees to open toward the wall.

3. Rest the hands on the belly, lay them out to the sides or overhead.

Remain in the posture 3-5 minutes

Benefits:	Cautions:
• Stretches the hips and groins	• Hip replacement • Groin injury

Tips/Variations:

- Blocks or rolled blankets may be placed under the knees for additional comfort.

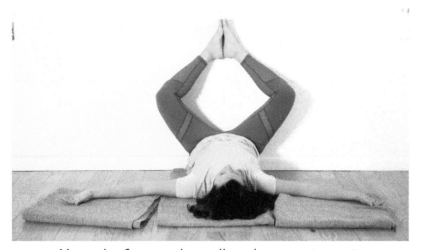

Move the feet up the wall to decrease intensity

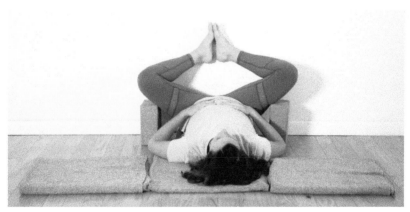

Blocks can be used to support the legs

Section 4

Assists

Assists in restorative yoga are used to help students release and find space and comfort. Find the angles in your own body that are most comfortable for you to transmit to the receiver. Developing a keen eye takes practice and tutelage from an experienced restorative trainer. Look to see where the body is holding tension and help the client breathe into that space.

Assisting is an additional art form. Additional training in assisting techniques should be a part of a teacher's continuing education. When in doubt, keep hands-off. Be sure to understand the scope of your practice and operate under the applicable rules and laws. For example you are not a massage therapist or physical therapist unless you have completed your licensing in those areas.

On the following pages are some examples of assists. Many can be used beyond the pose that they are being shown with. Be creative; find new poses to use the assists. Look for other ways to help a student find deeper stretch and greater ease within a pose.

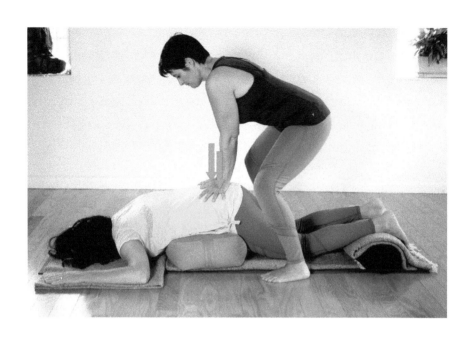

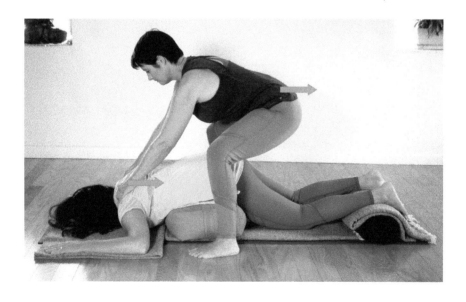

216

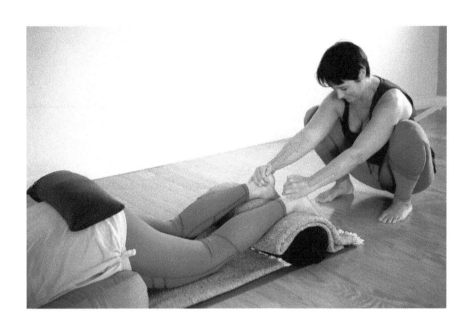

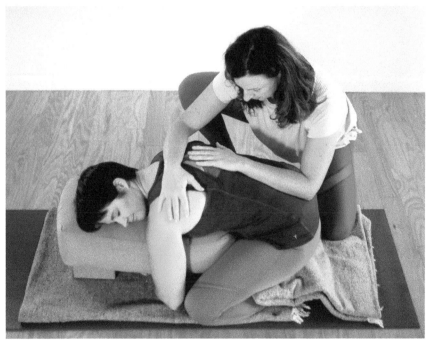

place arms on the back body. encouraging students to breath into the back

217

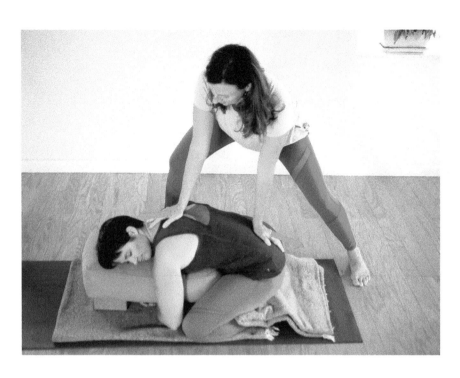

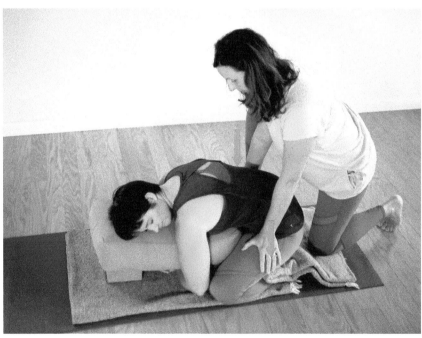

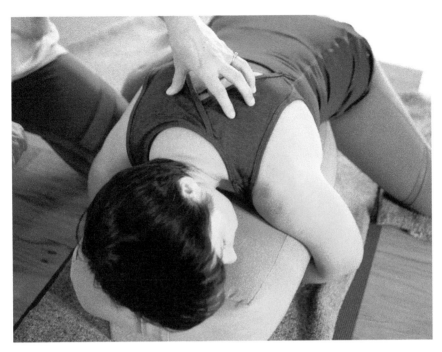

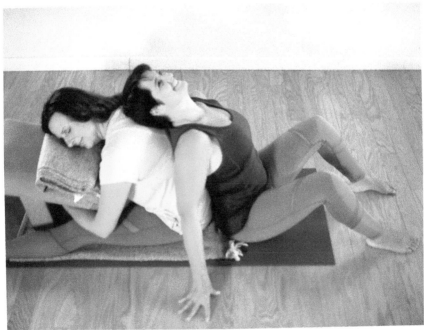

Feels great for both the giver and receiver

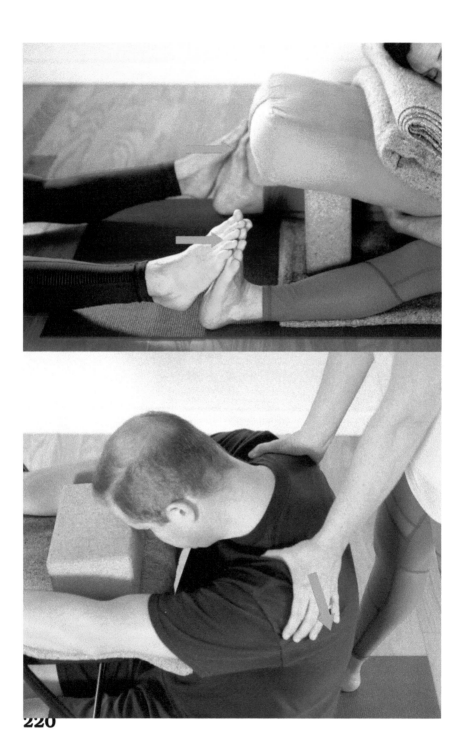

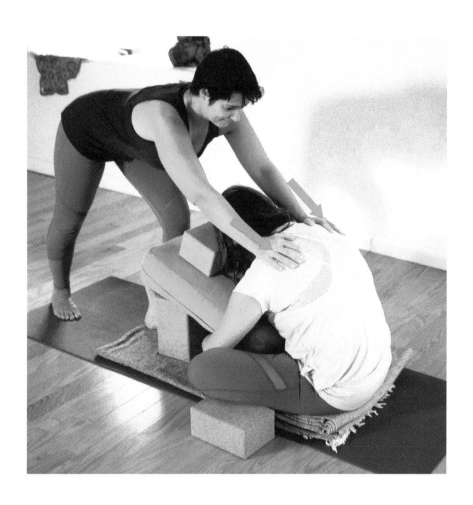

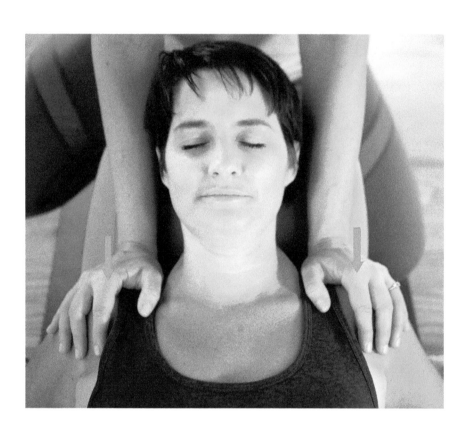

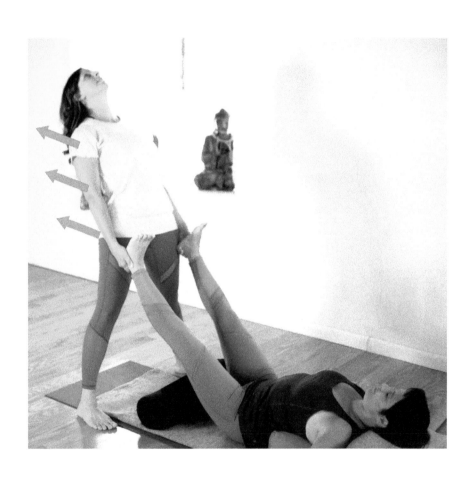

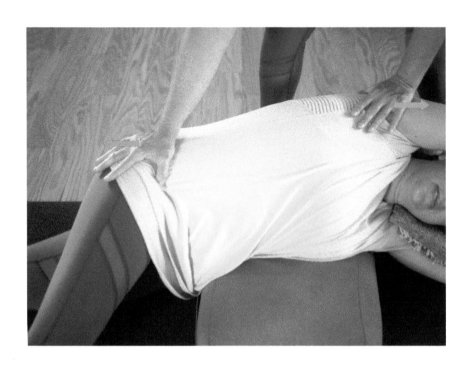

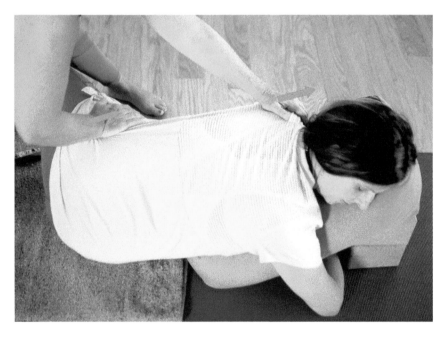

224

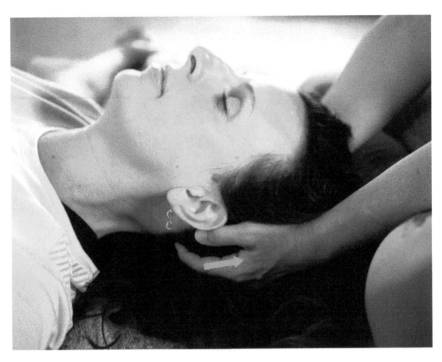

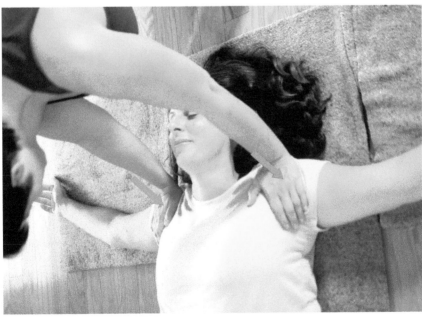

225

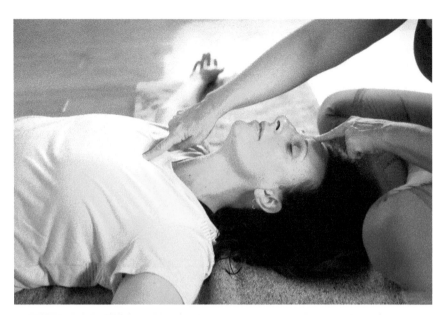

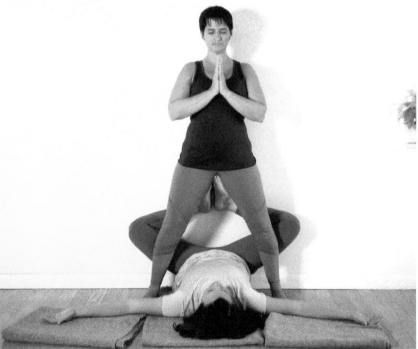

Gently straighten the legs to push the receiver's legs toward the wall

226

Section 5

Subtle Energy: Hands Off/Hands On

"Everything turns in circles and spirals with the cosmic heart until infinity. Everything has a vibration that spirals inward or outward — and everything turns together in the same direction at the same time. This vibration keeps going: it becomes born and expands or closes and destructs — only to repeat the cycle again in opposite current. Like a lotus, it opens or closes, dies and is born again. Such is also the story of the sun and moon, of me and you. Nothing truly dies. All energy simply transforms." - **Suzy Kassem, Rise Up and Salute the Sun: The Writings of Suzy Kassem**

Introduction to Subtle Energy

What are energy fields? Why do you need to know anything about them?

Prana is a Sanskrit word which is difficult to translate directly, since it encompasses a variety of ideas and concepts. Essentially, it would be taken to mean "energy" or "life force," but these definitions do not quite do justice to the word. *Prana* is also associated with breath, although air itself is not *prana*; rather, breathing can be used to focus and control *prana* as part of a spiritual practice. (*Chi* is the equivalent force in Traditional Chinese Medicine aka TCM)

Nadis: 72,000 psychic channels (Similar to Meridians in TCM and *Sen* Lines in Thai Massage)

Nerve Impulses are Electricity in the Body

Nerve impulses travel through the nervous system and brain and are human electricity created by chemical processes in the body. The nervous system is a network of billions of nerve cells called neurons with around 100 billion neurons in the brain itself. Your body has nerves for movement, brain-nerves for thinking, and nerves of feeling which go to all parts of the outer body. In effect, we have a complete human electrical system throughout the body.

We are electrical beings at the physical level so we can pass on, pick up, and feel the electrical and magnetic fields of others. As electricity passes through a metal wire it causes an energy field or magnetic field. In similar ways human electricity in nerves create a human magnetic field around the nerves. The millions of nerve impulses in the body create complex human magnetic fields. The heart creates the largest human energy field which can be measured by instruments. The nervous system can create human electric energy waves that can be measured with scientific instruments.

Kundalini, the Subtle Bodies and the Chakras

Kundalini is a Sanskrit word for "Corporeal Energy." *Kundalini* is often described as the potential force waiting to be awakened in each of us. India tradition uses the visual of a sleeping serpent coiled three and a half time at the base of the sacrum. Each coil represents one of the *gunas (sattva, raja, tamas)*, while the last half coil signifies transcendence. This dormant force/energy/potential is "awakened" through various techniques including *pranayama, asana*, meditation and *mantras*. When *Kundalini* is activated, the power of it is said to include extreme physical sensation, visions, brilliant lights, bliss, ecstasy, and extreme clarity. Some schools believe that it is so powerful that it should only be awakened under the guidance of a teacher so that the movement doesn't rise too quickly and cause the practitioner alarm or harm.

Another way of describing the rise of *Kundalini* is that the *Shakti* (feminine aspect) rises on *Kundalini* (the vehicle) to unite with *Shiva* (masculine aspect). When both masculine and feminine

230

aspects unite the body comes into balance and is open to higher expression.

Chakra is a Sanskrit word meaning "Wheel". It refers to the belief, in traditional Indian medicine, that there are energy vortices spinning in the body. These force centers in the subtle body rise from a point in the physical body and are considered to be focal points for the reception and transmission of energy.[3] Different systems cite different amount of *chakras*. Seven main *chakras* are usually referred to: *muladhara* the root *chakra*, *svadhisthana* the sacral *chakra*, *manipura* the solar plexus *chakra*, *anahata* the heart *chakra*, *visuddha* the throat *chakra*, *ajna* the third eye or brow *chakra*, and *sahasrara* the crown *chakra*. These seven *chakras* are associated with location, *mantra*, *Yantra*, element, gemstones, herbs, *mudra*, deities, emotions, and bodily functions.

The location of each of the seven *chakras* is where three of the main *nadis* (energy channels) cross. It is said that there are 72,000 psychic channels in the body. The three main channels are *Ida*, *Pingala*, and *Sushumna nadi*. All three *nadis* originate at the base of the coccyx. *Sushumna nadi* runs from the coccyx, just in front of the spine, to the crown of the head as the central channel for the rising of *Kundalini* energy. *Ida nadi* begins on the left while *pingala* starts on the right. *Ida* and *pingala* continually cross paths along *sushumna nadi* and each place they cross is where a *chakra* is centered. *Ida* is associated with the feminine aspect while *pingala* represents the masculine aspect.

─────────────

3 *Healing with the Chakra Energy System*, John Cross, Robert Charman pp. 17–18.

The *chakra* model is one way to paint a poetic and visual experience. Information and verbal adventures should be balanced with silence and space for students to settle and feel. There are many different yoga related models you may explore and the chakras are one of the more common tools for teachers.

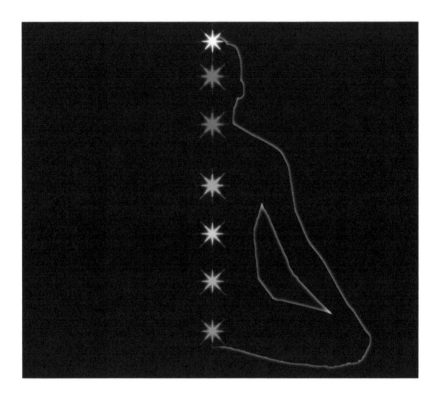

Root or *muladhara chakra*

Represents our foundation and feeling of being rooted and grounded.

Location	Base of spine/tailbone area. Pelvic floor area in restorative poses.
Emotion	Survival issues such as financial independence, money and food, and connection to family/tribe.
Color	Red
Under-activity	Apathy, weakness, depression, passivity, lethargy.

Sacral or *svadhisthana chakra*

Our connection and ability to accept others and new experiences.

Location	Lower abdomen, about two inches below the navel and two inches in.
Emotion	Sense of abundance, creativity, well-being, pleasure and sexuality.
Color	Orange
Under-activity	disinterest, repressed feelings, self-deprivation, depression, sexual repression.

Solar Plexus or *manipura chakra*

Our ability to be confident and in control of our lives.

Location	Upper abdomen in the navel area.
Emotion	Self-worth, self-confidence and self-esteem.
Color	Yellow
Under-activity	Indecisive, inability to concentrate, naive, passive, oblivious.

Heart or *anahata chakra*

Our ability to love and be loved.

Location	Center of chest just above the heart.
Emotion	Love, joy and inner peace.
Color	Green
Under-activity	Loneliness, neediness, greed jealousy, inability to love or be loved.

Throat or *visuddha chakra*

Our ability to communicate and be authentic.

Location	Throat
Emotion	Communication, self-expression of feelings and the truth.
Color	Blue
Under-activity	Dishonesty, repressed expression, over-conversational, gossipy, negative, preoccupation with others, gullibility.

Third eye or *ajna chakra*

Our ability to gain clarity and see truth.

Location	Forehead between the eyes
Emotion	Intuition, imagination, wisdom and the ability to think and make clear decisions.
Color	Indigo
Under-activity	Lack of imagination, insensitivity, self-absorption, narrow mind, Paranoia, daydreamer, tendency to space out.

Crown or *sahasrara chakra*

The highest chakra represents our ability to be fully connected spiritually.

Location	Forehead between the eyes
Emotion	Inner and outer beauty, our connection to spirituality (one might use God or Universe) and pure bliss or *samadhi*.
Color	Violet or White
Under-activity	Depression, lack of empathy, dizziness, mental fogginess, light sensitivities.

Section 6

Sequences

"A sequence works in a way a collection never can." -**George Murray**

General Relaxation Flow

Seated Wide Forward Fold

Child's Pose

Seated Forward Fold

Supported Head-to-Knee

Reclining Bound Angle

Side Lying to Twist

Legs up the Wall

Fish Pose

Meditation

"A cheerful frame of mind, reinforced by relaxation... is the medicine that puts all ghosts of fear on the run."

-George Mathew Adams

Circulation Flow

Seated pose of choice for Pranayama

Fish Pose

Supported Bridge Pose

Side Lying Twist Prone Variation

Half Moon

Legs up the Wall

Bent Knee Hip Opener

Mountain Brook

"If you want to cultivate a habit, do it without any reservation, till it is firmly established. Until it is so confirmed, until it becomes a part of your character, let there be no exception, no relaxation of effort."

- Mahavira

Flow for Digestion and Elimination

Hero's Pose or Half-Hero's Forward Fold

Cow Face Pose

Child's Pose

Side Lying Twist Supine Variation

Side Lying Twist Prone Variation

Legs Up The Wall

Reclining Bound Angle

Mountain Brook

"Life is a series of natural and spontaneous changes. Don't resist them - that only creates sorrow. Let reality be reality. Let things flow naturally forward in whatever way they like."

-Lao Tzu

De-stress Flow

Joint Mobility with some simple seated cat cow

Reclining Bound Angle

Half Hero's Forward Fold

Hero's pose- Pranayama (either 3 part breathing or Ujjayi)

Legs up the Wall

Inverted Reclining Bound Angle

Seated meditation

Fish Pose

"The greatest weapon against stress is our ability to choose one thought over another."

-William James

My Flows

"I will master something; then the creativity will come." -Japanese
Proverb

My Flows

"Creativity is the natural extension of your enthusiasm." -Earl Nightingale

My Flows

"Creativity is contagious, pass it on." -Albert Einstein

My Flows

"Passion is one great force that unleashes creativity, because if you're passionate about something, then you're more willing to take risks." -Yo Yo Ma

Section 7

Afterword

"If you could call it perfection, what would it look like? How would you know it? Would you feel it? Wherever you are now call it perfection and know in this moment it really is enough –**Liza Lowitz, Lines to Unfold By**

Chris on Inversions

There is some debate among certain schools as to if a student should or should not practice inversions during their menstrual cycles. Many yogic texts will cite energetic reasons not to do inversions, mainly due to apana, or the downward flow of elimination. Apana, however, is the energy of elimination and is multi-directional. When you exhale you are using the force of apana, and the exhale moves up and out of the lungs, vomiting also comes up before it goes down. We eliminate our bowels daily and yet we are told inversions are beneficial. One type of elimination is OK and not the other? With these questions in mind I checked in with 14 different members of the medical community and all of them agreed that there was no medical reason not to practice inversions during the menstrual cycle. The only reasonable advice they could offer was if you don't feel so well, rest (good advice in general).

I had been told for years by various teachers not to do inversions during my cycle and had avoided doing so. I decided after the doctor's advice to try some myself and make note of any sensational differences during my practice of inversions at that time. Much to my surprise, I found that my cramps would go away completely and more challenging inversions that I often struggled with seemed to effortlessly fall into place during my moon cycle.

Working with a group of acrobats and performers, I asked many women to join me in the experiment. The results for each of these women were strikingly similar. My future plan is to gain funding for a full scale study on the effects of inversions on menstruation.

From both doctors' advice and personal research, my belief is that the idea of apana and banning women from inversions came from a time when women's issues were largely misunderstood. A woman bleeding can be scary to a premedical community of men. I am sure it was with wise caution that they thought it might be best not to do anything. So I would offer that if it feels good to you, go ahead and invert and if you are feeling uncomfortable, then avoid them.

Many educators religiously cling to an idea because it came from their guru and/or the idea has been around for a long time. I invite you to question all things and investigate for yourself. If new information is more relevant, always be willing to change your mind. Agree or disagree, you will see me happily hanging out in my best handstand relieving my cramps and enjoying what feels right in my body.

Jessica on Reiki

Reiki is a Japanese technique for stress reduction and relaxation that also promotes healing. It is administered by "laying on hands" and is based on the idea that an unseen "life force energy" flows through us and is what causes us to be alive. If one's "life force energy" is low, then we are more likely to get sick or feel stress, and if it is high, we are more capable of being happy and healthy.

The word Reiki is made of two Japanese words - Rei which means "God's Wisdom or the Higher Power" and Ki which is "life force energy". So Reiki is actually "spiritually guided life force energy."

If you have not had training in Reiki, not to worry. If you move with intention towards the client's greatest and highest good, you can ask for divine energy to be brought to each person in your class. You cannot "hurt" another person in this manner. Trust that Reiki is happening through you if you are acting from a place of the highest good. Make sure to have proper Reiki training and an attunement before advertising this as part of your class experience. Reiki can be a great way of addressing imbalances in the chakras. Before administering Reiki, as a rule, first ask your students if they would like to receive Reiki. Students can place a prop at the top of their mat indicating a yes or no.

About the Authors

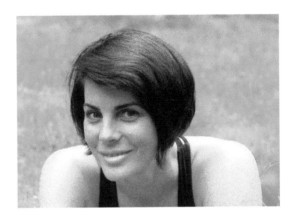

Chris

Chris Loebsack uses the power of yoga to create a space for students that cultivates trust, playfulness and Divine connection with themselves and with community. Living by her mantra, Clarity, Integrity and Love, she draws upon her partner yoga practice to share the healing power of touch and safe intimacy.

Chris is a full time teacher and owner of Boundless Yoga Studios in

Pennsylvania. Her playful yet focused classes are filled with user friendly gems of applied anatomy leaving students with a greater understanding of how to find comfort and space in their bodies and smiles beaming across their faces. She encourages teachers to set a higher standard of excellence through knowledge and has become a valuable mentor to many upcoming yoga educators.

500HR E.R.Y.T, Sundari Yoga 250, Dharma Yoga® 500, AcroYoga® L1&2 , AcroFit, ASFYT®, Zenyasa® 300, Restorative Yoga, Yin Yoga, Chair Yoga, Aerial Yoga and Thai Massage Certified L1-2-3, BA in Theater and Biology from East Stroudsburg University

www.BoundlessMotion.com

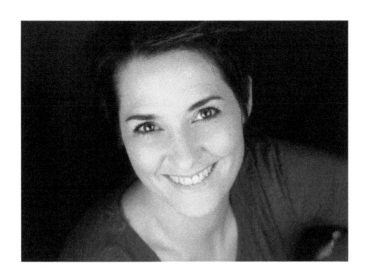

Tracy Gross

Tracy Gross, affectionately called Traé has a great appreciation for all forms of artistic expression. Featured as Annie on Broadway as a child star she stepped back to a quieter space settling in the Pocono Mountains, Pennsylvania. She uses her love of mixed media to create incredibly unique jewelry, teach yoga and run art as meditation workshops. Creativity breathes into every aspect of her being.

500HR E.R.Y.T, Boundless Restorative Yoga, Yin Yoga, Artist and Jewelry Designer and Reiki Master

www.TreaBeTrue.com

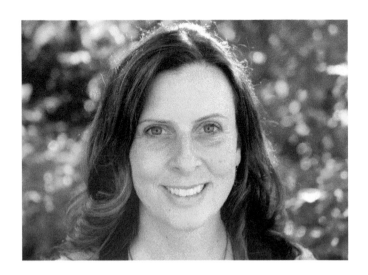

Jessica Batha

Jessica Batha combines her talents in movement, yoga, dance, massage, and aromatherapy to help others cultivate joy and space in their bodies and in their lives. Her dedication to her continued education is matched by her passion for sharing and nourishing others. She resides in Bangor, Pennsylvania with her amazing husband and two beautiful children.

500HR R.Y.T, Boundless Yoga 200, Boundless Yoga 300, Boundless Restorative Yoga, and Reiki Master, Adjunct Professor at Fairleigh Dickinson University and East Stroudsburg University (MFA-Dance)

www.AdoraSessions.com/

"Thanks for sharing so well. Chris you are amazing, and so selfless!!!" - Matt Giordano, AcroYoga® Instructor and Lululemon ambassador

Tracy was great: warm, friendly and professional! - Betsy

I love Restorative Flow on Sunday nights with you Tracy. It's the best part of my week. A complete reset for the week ahead. Thank you! - Jenn

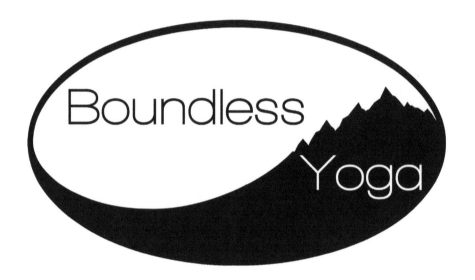